Feedback That Sticks

THE ART OF COMMUNICATING

NEUROPSYCHOLOGICAL ASSESSMENT RESULTS

Karen Postal and Kira Armstrong

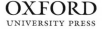

OXFORD

UNIVERSITY PRESS

OXFORD
UNIVERSITY PRESS

Oxford University Press is a department of the University of Oxford.
It furthers the University's objective of excellence in research, scholarship,
and education by publishing \worldwide.

Oxford   New York
Auckland   Cape Town   Dar es Salaam   Hong Kong   Karachi
Kuala Lumpur   Madrid   Melbourne   Mexico City   Nairobi
New Delhi   Shanghai   Taipei   Toronto

With offices in
Argentina   Austria   Brazil   Chile   Czech Republic   France   Greece
Guatemala   Hungary   Italy   Japan   Poland   Portugal   Singapore
South Korea   Switzerland   Thailand   Turkey   Ukraine   Vietnam

Copyright © 2013 by Oxford University Press

Published in the United States of America by
Oxford University Press
198 Madison Avenue, New York, NY 10016, United States of America
www.oup.com

Oxford is a registered trademark of Oxford University Press in the UK and
in certain other countries

Library of Congress Cataloging-in-Publication Data
Postal, Karen.
    Feedback that sticks : the art of communicating neuropsychological assessment results / Karen Postal and
    Kira Armstrong.
    p. cm.
    Includes bibliographical references and index.
    ISBN 978–0–19–976569–0 (alk. paper)
    1. Neuropsychology.   2. Feedback (Psychology)
    I. Armstrong, Kira.   II. Title.
    QP360.P67 2013
    616.8—dc23
    2012026696

To my husband, Bill Postal, and my children, Andrew, Robbie, and Caroline: love that sticks.

To my father, Verne Spangenberg, who taught me about strength of character, independence, and the love of a good book. Dad, you'll always be one of the good guys.

And to my first mentor in neuropsychology, Dr. Linda Vincent, who thought I might make a good neuropsychologist, and made some calls.

—Karen Postal

To my wonderful husband, Zack Armstrong, and my children, Aidan and Logan. Thank you for your ongoing support – and for patiently nodding your head every time I promised, "I'm done with the book – for real this time!"

And to everyone who has helped me learn how to make feedback stick – both my neuropsychological mentors and the patients and families who have shared their lives with me.

—Kira Armstrong

Table of Contents

Acknowledgments

WE WANT TO offer heartfelt thanks to Joan Bossert, our editor, who believed feedback was a subject whose time had come. We also want to thank our many colleagues who generously offered to sit down and share all of their best feedback techniques.

Contributors

Mark T. Barisa, Ph.D., ABPP/CN
Director of Neuropsychology Services,
   Baylor Institute for Rehabilitation,
   Dallas, Texas

William B. Barr, Ph.D., ABPP/CN
Departments of Neurology and Psychiatry,
   New York University School of Medicine

John T. Beetar, PhD, ABPP/CN
Kennedy Krieger Institute, Johns Hopkins
   University School of Medicine,
   Baltimore, Maryland

Erin D. Bigler, Ph.D., ABPP/CN
Professor of Psychology and Neuroscience,
   Brigham Young University, Salt Lake
   City, Utah

Robert M. Bilder, Ph.D., ABPP/CN
Michael E. Tennenbaum Family Professor
   of Psychiatry and Biobehavioral
   Sciences, David Geffen School of
   Medicine at UCLA
Professor of Psychology, UCLA College of
   Letters and Science
Chief of Medical
   Psychology-Neuropsychology, Semel
   Institute for Neuroscience and
   Human Behavior, and Stewart and
   Lynda Resnick Neuropsychiatric
   Hospital

Julie Bobholtz, Ph.D., ABPP/CN
Associate Clinical Professor, Department
   of Neurology, Medical College of
   Wisconsin

Thomas Boll, Ph.D., ABPP/CN
Director, Neuropsychology Institute,
  Birmingham, Alabama

Mark W. Bondi, Ph.D., ABPP/CN
Professor of Psychiatry, University
  of California San Diego School of
  Medicine
Director, Neuropsychological Assessment
  Unit, VA San Diego Healthcare
  System

Katrina Boyer, Ph.D.
Director, Neuropsychology of Epilepsy
  Program, Division of Epilepsy and
  Clinical Neurophysiology, Children's
  Hospital, Boston

Anne Bradley, Ph.D.
Roger C. Peace Rehabilitation Hospital,
  Greenville, South Carolina

Dominic A. Carone, Ph.D., ABPP/CN
SUNY Upstate Medical University,
  Syracuse, New York

Gordon J. Chelune, Ph.D., ABPP/CN
Head, Section of Clinical
  Neuropsychology, Professor, Department
  of Neurology, Center for Alzheimer
  Care, Imaging and Research, University
  of Utah

Roger Cohen, Ph.D.
Independent Practice, Boston,
  Massachusetts

Jeff Cory, Ph.D.
Independent Practice, Bozeman, Montana
Adjunct Professor, Washington Wyoming
  Alaska Montana and Idaho (WWAMI)
  Medical Program, Montana State
  University and University of Washington
  School of Medicine

Paul L. Craig, Ph.D., ABPP/CN
Independent Practice, Anchorage, Alaska
Clinical Professor, WWAMI Program,
  Department of Psychiatry and Behavioral
  Sciences, University of Washington
  School of Medicine

C. Munro Cullum, Ph.D., ABPP/CN
Professor of Psychiatry, Professor of
  Neurology and Neurotherapeutics, Pam
  Blumenthal Distinguished Professor of
  Clinical Psychology
Director, Neuropsychology, The University
  of Texas Southwestern Medical Center
  at Dallas

**Robert L. Denney, Psy.D., ABPP/CN,
ABFP**
School of Professional Psychology at the
  Forrest Institute and The U.S. Medical
  Center for Federal Prisoners, Springfield,
  Missouri

Jacobus Donders, Ph.D., ABPP/CN
Chief Psychologist, Mary Free Bed
  Rehabilitation Hospital, Grand Rapids,
  Michigan

Deborah Fein, Ph.D.
University of Connecticut Board of
  Trustees Distinguished Professor,
  Department of Psychology, Department
  of Pediatrics, University of Connecticut

Tanis J. Ferman, Ph.D., ABPP/CN
The University of Texas Southwestern
  Medical Center at Dallas, Texas

Judith M. Glasser, Ph.D.
Independent Practice, Silver Spring,
  Maryland

Ketty Patiño González, Ph.D.
Independent Practice, Coral Gables, Florida

Gail M. Grodzinsky, Ph.D., ABPP/CN
Staff Neuropsychologist, Department of
  Psychiatry, Children's Hospital, Boston
Independent Practice, Lexington,
  Massachusetts

Christopher Grote, Ph.D., ABPP/CN
Professor, Associate Chair, Director of
  Neuropsychology, Department of
  Behavioral Sciences, Rush University
  Medical Center
Chicago, Illinois

Steven C. Guy, Ph.D.
Pediatric Neuropsychologist, Columbus, Ohio

James B. Hale, Ph.D., ABPdN
Associate Professor of Clinical
  Neuropsychology, University of Victoria,
  Wellington, Australia

Robin Hanks, Ph.D., ABPP-CN
Chief of Rehabilitation Psychology and
  Neuropsychology, Director of Training
  in Clinical Neuropsychology, Wayne
  State University Physician Group and
  Rehabilitation Institute of Michigan,
  Associate Professor, Wayne State University
  School of Medicine, Detroit, Michigan

Robert L. Heilbronner, Ph.D., ABPP/CN
Independent Practice, The Chicago
  Neuropsychology Group, Chicago, Illinois

Winifred Hentschel, Ed.D.
Independent Practice, Cambridge,
  Massachusetts

Robin C. Hilsabeck, Ph.D., ABPP/CN
Associate Professor, Department of
  Psychiatry, University of Texas Health
  Science Center at San Antonio

Steve Hughes, Ph.D., ABPdN
Independent Practice, St. Paul, Minnesota

James W. Irby, Jr., Ph.D., ABPP/CN
Clinical Neuropsychologist, Methodist
  Rehabilitation Center, Jackson,
  Mississippi

Jennifer Janusz, Psy.D., ABPP/CN
Children's Hospital Colorado,
  Assistant Professor of Pediatrics,
  University of Colorado Denver School
  of Medicine

Laura Janzen, Ph.D., ABPP/CN
The Hospital for Sick Children, Toronto,
  Ontario, Canada

Michael Joschko, Ph.D.
Senior Psychologist, Queen Alexandra
  Centre for Children's Health, Victoria,
  British Columbia

Paul Kaufmann, JD, Ph.D., ABPP/CN
University of Oregon, Eugene, Oregon

Julie Keaveney, Psy.D.
Independent Practice, Pennsylvania and
  Delaware

John W. Kirk, Psy.D., ABPP/CN
Children's Hospital, Colorado, Aurora,
  Colorado

Michael W. Kirkwood, Ph.D., ABPP/CN
Department of Physical Medicine and
  Rehabilitation, Children's Hospital
  Colorado, University of Colorado
  School of Medicine

Cynthia S. Kubu, Ph.D., ABPP/CN
Center for Neurological Restoration,
  Cleveland Clinic

Greg J. Lamberty, Ph.D., ABPP/CN
Rehabilitation/EC&R Psychology
  Supervisor, Clinical Neuropsychology
  Postdoctoral Fellowship, Minneapolis
  VA Health Care System, Minnesota

Gregory P. Lee, Ph.D., ABPP/CN
Department of Neurology, Medical College
  of Georgia, Georgia Health Sciences
  University, Augusta

Cynthia Levinson, Ph.D.
Independent Practice, Braintree,
  Massachusetts

Muriel D. Lezak, Ph.D.
Emeritus Professor of Neurology, Oregon
  Health Sciences University

John A. Lucas, Ph.D., ABPP/CN
Professor of Psychology, Chair Division
  of Psychology, Mayo Clinic, Rochester,
  Minnesota

**William S. MacAllister, Ph.D., ABPP/
CN**
New York University School of
  Medicine, Department of Neurology,
  Comprehensive Epilepsy Center

Karin JM McCoy, Ph.D., ABPP/CN
South Texas Veterans Health Care System
  and University of Texas Health Science
  Center at San Antonio

E. Mark Mahone, Ph.D., ABPP/CN
Director of Neuropsychology, Kennedy
  Krieger Institute, Associate Professor
  of Psychiatry and Behavioral Sciences,
  Johns Hopkins School of Medicine

Robb Mapou, Ph.D., ABPP/CN
Independent Practice, The Stixrud Group,
  Silver Spring, Maryland

**Bernice A. Marcopulos, Ph.D., ABPP/
CN**
Associate Professor, Department of
  Graduate Psychology, James Madison
  University, Harrisonburg, Virginia

Michael McCrea, Ph.D., ABPP/CN
Professor and Director of Brain Injury
  Research, Departments of Neurosurgery
  and Neurology, Medical College of
  Wisconsin, Wauwatosa, Wisconsin

Susan McPherson, Ph.D., ABPP/CN, LP
Associate Professor of Neurology,
  University of Minnesota School of
  Medicine
Private Practice, Edina, Minnesota

Monica Rivera Mindt, Ph.D.
Associate Professor, Department of
  Psychology, Fordham University, New
  York

Joel E. Morgan, Ph.D., ABPP/CN
Independent Practice, Madison, NJ
Department of Neurology, New Jersey
  Medical School, Newark, New Jersey

Richard Naugle, Ph.D., ABPP/CN
Head, Neuropsychology Section
  Neurological Institute, Cleveland Clinic,
  Ohio

Aaron Nelson, Ph.D., ABPP/CN
Chief of Psychology and Behavioral
  Neurology, Brigham and Women's
  Hospital, Boston
Assistant Professor, Harvard Medical
  School, Cambridge, Massachusetts

**Christopher Nicholls, Ph.D., ABPP/CL,
ABPdN**
Independent Practice, Scottsdale, Arizona

Marc A. Norman, Ph.D., ABPP/CN
Professor, Department of Psychiatry,
Director of the Neuropsychiatry/
Epilepsy Clinical Evaluation Program,
University of California, San Diego

Margaret O'Connor, Ph.D., ABPP/CN
Director of Neuropsychology, Department
of Neurology, Beth Israel Deaconess
Medical Center
Associate Professor of Neurology,
Harvard Medical School, Cambridge,
Massachusetts

Keith Owen Yeates, Ph.D., ABPP/CN
Department of Pediatrics, The Ohio State
University, Department of Psychology,
Nationwide Children's Hospital,
Columbus, Ohio

**Edward A. "Ted" Peck III, PhD., ABPP/
CN**
Independent Practice, Richmond, Virginia

Jennifer Turek Queally, PhD
Children's Hospital, Boston, Massachusetts

**Christopher Randolph, Ph.D., ABPP/
CN**
Clinical Professor of Neurology, Director
Neuropsychology Service, Loyola
University Medical Center, Proviso,
Illinois

John J. Randolph, Ph.D., ABPP/CN
Independent Practice, Lebanon, New
Hampshire

Lisa Riemenschneider, Psy.D.
Delnor/Central DuPage Hospital,
Winfield, Illinois

Joseph H. Ricker, Ph.D., ABPP/CN, RP
Department of Physical Medicine and
Rehabilitation, University of Pittsburgh
School of Medicine

Joel Rosenbaum, Ph.D.
Independent Practice, Boston,
Massachusetts

Beth Rush, Ph.D., ABPP/CN, RP
Mayo Clinic, Florida

Laurie M. Ryan, Ph.D.
National Institutes of Health*, Bethesda,
Maryland

**Michael P. Santa Maria, Ph.D.,
ABPP/CN**
DeGraff Hospital

Jim Scott, Ph.D., ABPP/CN
Professor, Oklahoma University Health
Sciences Center (OUHSC College of
Medicine ,Oklahoma City, Oklahoma
Clinical Neuropsychologist, Department of
Psychiatry and Behavioral Sciences

Marla B. Shapiro, Ph.D.
Independent Practice, Rockville,
Maryland

Barbara J. Schrock, Ph.D., ABPP/CN
Lead Clinical Neuropsychologist,
Sharp HealthCare, San Diego,
California

Hillary Shurtleff, Ph.D., ABPP/CN
Department of Neurology, Washington
School of Medicine
Department of Psychiatry, Seattle
Children's Hospital

*Dr. Ryan contributed to this book in her personal capacity. The views expressed are her own and do not necessarily represent the views of the National Institutes of Health or the United States Government.

Brenda J. Spiegler, Ph.D., ABPP/CN
Director, Department of Psychology,
  Hospital for Sick Children
Associate Professor, Faculty of Medicine,
  University of Toronto, Toronto, Ontario

Janine Stasior, PhD., M.S., ABPdN
Child Development Network, Lexington,
  Massachusetts

Yana Suchy, Ph.D.
Associate Professor, Department of
  Psychology, University of Utah, Salt
  Lake City, Utah

Sara J. Swanson, Ph.D., ABPP/CN
Professor, Department of Neurology,
  Medical Center of Wisconsin,
  Milwaukee, Wisconsin

H. Gerry Taylor, Ph.D., ABPP/CN
Professor of Pediatrics, Case Western
  Reserve University, Rainbow Babies and
  Children's Hospital, University Hospitals
  Medical Center

David E. Tupper, Ph.D.
Director, Neuropsychology Section,
  Hennepin County Medical Center,
  Minneapolis, Minnesota

Linda Vincent, Ph.D.
Independent Practice, Northampton,
  Massachusetts

Deborah P. Waber, Ph.D.
Senior Associate, Department of Psychiatry,
  Children's Hospital, Boston
Director, Learning Disabilities Program,
  Department of Neurology, Children's
  Hospital, Boston
Associate Professor, Department of
  Psychiatry, Harvard Medical School,
  Cambridge, Massachusetts

Mary (Molly) Warner, Ph.D., ABPP/CN
Epilepsy and Epilepsy Surgery Program,
  Seattle Children's Hospital,
  Washington

Cheryl Weinstein Ph.D., ABPP/CN
Assistant Professor of Clinical
  Psychology, Harvard Medical School,
  Beth Israel Deaconess Medical Center,
  Longwood Neuropsychology Training
  Program, Cambridge and Boston,
  Massachusetts

Michael Westerveld, Ph.D., ABPP/CN
Medical Director, Pediatric
  Neuropsychology, Walt Disney Pavilion,
  Florida Hospital for Children, Orlando,
  Florida

Desirée A. White, Ph.D.
Associate Professor, Department of
  Psychology, Washington University in St.
  Louis, Missouri

Roberta F. White, Ph.D.
Professor and Chair, Department of
  Environmental Health
Associate Dean for Research, Boston
  University School of Public Health

Karen E. Wills, Ph.D., LP., ABPP/CN
Children's Hospitals and Clinics of
  Minnesota, Minneapolis,
  Minnesota

Rebecca Wilson, Psy.D.
Lead Psychologist, Child Development
  Unit
Assistant Professor,
  Neurodevelopmental-Behavioral
  Pediatrics and Psychiatry
University of Colorado School of
  Medicine, Aurora,
  Colorado

Tony Wong,[†] **Ph.D., ABPP/CN**
Department of Physical Medicine and
  Rehabilitation
University of Rochester Medical Center
Department of Neuropsychology
Unity Health System, Rochester, NY

Keith Owen Yeates, Ph.D., ABPP/CN
Department of Pediatrics, The Ohio State
  University
Department of Psychology, Nationwide
  Children's Hospital, Columbus, Ohio

T. Andrew Zabel, Ph.D., ABPP/CN
Department of Neuropsychology, Kennedy
  Krieger Institute
Department of Psychiatry and Behavioral
  Science, Johns Hopkins University
  School of Medicine, Baltimore,
  Maryland

Andrea L. Zartman, Ph.D., ABPP/CN
VA North Texas Health Care System,
  Dallas, Texas

Prologue

IN RESEARCHING THIS book we had the unique pleasure and opportunity to sit with over 85 of our colleagues for in-depth interviews. We started with the premise that explaining complex neuropsychological assessment results to cognitively impaired patients and their families is a very difficult task; and that seasoned clinicians have created, stumbled upon, or inherited ways of explaining clinical phenomena and findings that engage patients in a way that can alter lives. In order to find these "pearls," we asked our colleagues to allow us to be "a fly on their office wall" as they provided feedback to their patients, and tell us verbatim what they say, and how they say it.

We found that the process of collecting clinical pearls was much like a treasure hunt. We searched widely, interviewing clinicians who work across the lifespan with diverse patient populations and in varying clinical settings. We conducted interviews at each neuropsychological conference over the course of 18 months, and issued invitations as widely as possible to neuropsychologists we knew would be attending the meetings or presenting their own research. We also opened a website to elicit feedback strategies from the larger neuropsychology community. It was striking that most interviews began with the same assertion, "I'm flattered you asked, but I don't have any pearls for you." Despite these reservations, over the course of each interview, a recollection of a patient or a question about a particular syndrome would trigger a pearl. And it was clear when one dropped onto the table between us. Then the analogies and strategies began to flow, triggering questions that generated more pearls. While transcribing our interviews we often laughed as we heard our own "Ooohs! and Ahhs!" as well as our pledges to grab *that one* right away for our own feedback sessions. At the end of these engaging and tangential dialogues, it typically seemed that, given enough time, we could have gathered several more baskets of pearls from every interviewee.

Some of the pearls we collected were created by our interviewees; others were inherited. Like all good folklore, many times the original author of a metaphor was uncertain: "I know I picked this one up while training, but I can't remember who said it!" When the lineage was known, it was often fascinating to hear it detailed: "That came from my post-doc supervisor, who heard it from his mentor.... " As we present the pearls throughout the book, we give credit to the clinicians who shared them, regardless of whether they were the original "authors." Similarly, we frequently heard the same pearl from many clinicians, often by people who had no common training or employment experiences, suggesting that some pearls have been created and recreated numerous times. In these instances we gave credit to the contributor who shared the metaphor first, or who presented it in the most compelling manner.

Like the spoils of a treasure hunt, our take was necessarily uneven. In following our interviewees (rather than leading them), we collected strategies pertinent to many clinical domains, and came up empty-handed for other topic areas. Had we sat down and manufactured pearls on our own, or conducted more restrictive, linear interviews, we might have been able to remedy the unevenness across clinical syndromes, but at the cost of much of the brilliance. You just can't make these up. We hope that this book represents the beginning of a larger treasure hunt to collect feedback pearls from every corner of our extraordinary field. Should your own pearls be triggered while reading this book, we have left our website open (http://www.karenpostal.com/feedback-that-sticks/) and welcome additional contributions for future editions.

Throughout the book, whether presenting pearls, general strategies, or social pragmatics of delivery, our purpose is the same. We are not attempting to describe what *should* be done, but rather to present the reader with an opportunity to "listen in on" a wide variety of pearls and strategies, as well as their rationales. By doing so, we hope to help equip clinicians with an arsenal of tools to deliver the type of striking feedback that alters lives.

While this book is one that we would have loved to read during our training, as seasoned clinicians we can testify that the process of listening in on the feedback techniques of over 85 preeminent colleagues has dramatically improved our own feedback styles. In fact, we both found ourselves regularly integrating pearls we gathered for the book: at first gingerly, and then with conviction, as we made them our own. We hope that seasoned clinicians will also use this book to add to their craft, and we encourage readers to explore the entire book, rather than focusing exclusively on their own clinical populations. We found ourselves integrating pearls into our clinical practices even if the original purpose was to explain a topic outside of our expertise.

Of course, the difficult task of engaging in hard conversations when treating patients with neurocognitive syndromes is shared with many other professions. Neurologists, clinical psychologists, pediatricians, family practitioners, social workers, psychiatrists, school psychologists, and many others may find the processes and pearls in this book helpful in their own interactions with patients/clients and their families. We hope this book can serve as a direct resource for our allied health professionals as well as a way to highlight the benefits of referring to neuropsychologists.

ORIENTATION TO THE REST OF THE BOOK

This book is divided into three parts. Part I explores the feedback process itself. The first two chapters address the fundamental questions—What is feedback? Why is feedback important? And what makes some feedback messages compelling and memorable? Chapters 3 and 4 present a variety of strategies for structuring feedback sessions, addressing how we set the stage for effective feedback—and just as important, how the words are delivered. We cover topics ranging from who is invited to our feedback sessions, to the social pragmatics of delivering feedback messages. Part II is devoted to the presentation of the pearls we collected—that is, the quotes, metaphors, and user-friendly explanations that clinicians use to convey complicated information to our patients. The first chapter in this section is devoted to pearls that are easily applied across multiple patient populations. The remaining chapters present pearls that are organized by neuropsychological syndrome. While these pearls were created for certain patient populations, many can be modified to fit a variety of populations. We therefore encourage readers to explore beyond their typical patient populations while reading the book. The final section of this book, Part III, addresses feedback to other professionals, as well as a brief overview of concepts and considerations for writing neuropsychological reports.

DISCLAIMER

The pearls and comments that are shared in this book are offered as vignettes, examples of how information is shared with patients, sometimes based on very specific clinical details. They may not always be appropriate to use, depending on the patient's neuropsychological and/or medical history. Some quotes also represent the personal opinions of neuropsychologists and may not be empirically supported.

KEY

Pearls are denoted in the text by the following symbol: o

I What Is Feedback, and What Makes It Stick?

1 Feedback That Sticks
THE ART OF COMMUNICATING NEUROPSYCHOLOGICAL ASSESSMENT RESULTS

THIS BOOK IS about how to give outstanding feedback to patients, their family members, and other professionals. Along with their neuropsychological syndromes, patients bring their personal histories, complex psychological presentations, and unique sociocultural backgrounds into our offices, seeking explanations for their presenting problems. The results are often unpredictable and require us to employ all of the expertise we have developed throughout our training and careers.

> *Feedback is the most integrated thing that we do. It brings together all of our knowledge and all of our training from every aspect of being a psychologist and neuropsychologist. We draw just as much from everything we've learned about human development, psychopathology, family systems, social psychology, social power theory, leadership, psychometrics—as well as neuroscience and the brain.*
> —*E. Mark Mahone, Ph.D.*

Even with this expertise, there are some things in a feedback session you simply cannot plan for:

> *I was giving feedback to an elderly man with a delusional misidentification syndrome that included the belief that there was an exact copy of his wife living with him. The patient came to the session with "that nice lady who is pretending to be my wife," and his son, a university professor. After hearing about his father's early dementia, the son brought up the issue of guns. I was surprised. "What guns?" The patient turned out to be a gun collector and had tons of guns around the house. All loaded. So I turn to the patient and ask him, "Well, what do you think about keeping the guns?" The patient admits, "Maybe it's not a good idea." Then the son asks, "But what about Mom's guns?" At that moment, all eyes turn to Mom as she clutches her handbag. It turns out that this elderly woman was licensed to carry concealed weapons!*

> *What are we going to say in feedback? I don't know. I'll find out when we get there. You have to meet people where they live. If I go into the feedback session, thinking, "I'm going to say this, and this and this..." Then you've lost them at hello.*
> —*Mark Barisa, Ph.D.*

WHY GIVE FEEDBACK?

Historically, a neuropsychologist's role was to provide succinct data on lesion location or the presence or absence of brain damage. Feedback was typically provided to referring physicians in the form of a report, rather than to patients face-to-face. Development of neuroimaging techniques, however, has shifted the identity of the field from that of "lesion location" to "what is the meaning of this lesion for the patient?" and to the identification of complex developmental and degenerative processes not easily captured through imaging technology. This shift in focus and increasing complexity of findings is reflected in an ever-growing percentage of neuropsychologists regularly providing direct patient feedback. Recent surveys (Pegg et al., 2008) have shown that the overwhelming majority of neuropsychologists (71%) in clinical practice now conduct feedback sessions with patients.

I have seen a big change in the course of my 31 years of practice. In the beginning, almost no patients requested feedback; now almost everyone does.
—*Roberta F. White, Ph.D.*

Cultural shifts in healthcare have also contributed to the establishment of feedback sessions as the norm rather than the exception. Over the past few decades, standards have changed for communication in general between doctors of all specialties and their patients. Paternalistic relationships have been replaced with collaborative relationships. Patients now expect to have their health conditions fully explained to them; the idea that professionals might communicate only amongst themselves feels alien to many health care consumers.

A growing body of research across medical specialties further indicates that when patients and caregivers understand their medical conditions, outcomes improve. In other words, this trend is not just a cultural shift towards greater patient–doctor collaboration: the collaboration itself has been shown to produce better outcomes. Communicating complex neuropsychological assessment results to patients who are cognitively impaired, however, is a significant challenge. Each patient has, by definition, his or her own unique capacity to understand and *misunderstand* our results. Therefore, the fundamental questions each neuropsychologist must ask include: Does the patient understand the findings? Will he or she remember them?

This difficulty in grasping complex neuropsychological assessment results might appear to offer a rationale for keeping the conversation about patients' cognitive conditions amongst medical professionals. However, Phillip Pegg and his team from the Virginia Commonwealth University found that direct communication of health information to patients with clear cognitive impairment, such as traumatic brain injury, significantly improved treatment outcomes, including the patients' effort in therapy and gains in functional independence (Pegg et. al., 2008). Furthermore, this very complexity means that neuropsychologists are often the only professionals capable of fully discussing their assessment findings with patients.

The neuropsychologist is in the best position to interpret data and communicate this to the family. I work with a great group of physicians. They know physical medicine and rehabilitation or transplants better than I do. And I know neuropsychology better than they do. I have never had anyone fight me on giving feedback about my assessment results directly to the patients. Down to a person, the physicians welcome me giving the neuropsychological feedback.
—*Joseph H. Ricker, Ph.D.*

In fact, many argue that providing direct feedback to patients should be considered a key element of a neuropsychologist's professional scope.

I am the attending neuropsychologist. I am in the best position to understand the test results themselves, interpret them clinically, and present them in a way the patient is able to incorporate them into their care plan. I do not see neuropsychology as a radiology model—where the physician interprets our results to patients.
—*Michael McCrea, Ph.D.*

WHAT IS FEEDBACK?

While interviewing neuropsychologists for this book, we discovered that many clinicians instinctively define "feedback" as the sharing of a patient's diagnosis. In a hospital setting, this definition can significantly limit the scope of a neuropsychologist's practice. For example, transplant teams, memory disorders clinics, or consult liaison services might designate neurologists or other physicians, rather than neuropsychologists, as the team members who give "the ultimate feedback." Given this assumption, many clinicians initially suggested they would not have much to offer for this book, because their clinical role did not include a discussion of the team's diagnostic impressions and conclusions. However, we (and they) soon discovered that in fact, these neuropsychologists provide a great deal of relevant, essential feedback, beyond the "punchline diagnosis" to the patients and families they see. This highlights a very critical point: Feedback sessions are not (just) about diagnoses. In fact, in some cases where a diagnosis is already known (e.g., following a traumatic brain injury [TBI], or treatment for a brain tumor), feedback sessions have very little to do with a label or identification of etiology.

Even when the provision of a diagnosis is a primary feature of the feedback session, Mark Barisa and Muriel Lezak remind us that the cost–benefit ratio of a two- to six-hour neuropsychological assessment is not really justified by "just" getting a diagnosis. We need to consider the value of our service and what it is we have to offer:

> *What is the patients' return on investment—what else could they have gotten with the time they put into the assessment? Will they find a 15-minute "Diagnose and Adios" session was worth all that time? If all they leave with is a diagnosis, then whoop-de-$%^!-do!*
>
> —Mark Barisa, Ph.D.

> *It's immoral to put a person through this kind of examination and not let them know how they did. I call it a hit and run assessment. There are always recommendations to be made. Sometimes the recommendation is only, "Hey, you're doing fine and keep doing what you're doing." But usually there's a lot more.*
>
> —Muriel D. Lezak, Ph.D.

While diagnoses are not considered the only, or even the most important aspect of a feedback session, neither are test scores. Indeed, the communication of scores was typically far down on the list of goals for the feedback session. Some clinicians shared that they avoid mentioning specific scores at all.

> *I personally think patients get almost nothing out of test scores. Scores are things patients seize upon without the tools to understand what the scores mean. It's hard enough to get our trainees to understand the scores, much less someone who just comes in for an assessment. No one really needs to know their score discrepancy—or what confidence interval we put around their memory quotient.*
>
> —Robert M. Bilder, Ph.D.

Or, put more succinctly,

> *I'm there to talk about the person—not the tests.*
>
> —*Christopher J. Nicholls, Ph.D.*

So, if not to provide patients with their scores or diagnosis, what is the purpose of feedback? Feedback is much more than a competent exchange of medical diagnoses and associated information. It is a comprehensive and

> *...clinical enterprise. And that's why we are trained as clinical psychologists. We can really shine with our knowledge base. We do a lot of education. But the point isn't just to give something a name.*
>
> —*Roberta F. White, Ph.D.*

> *We're the translators for the medical profession. We're the ones who are bridging the brain to behavior. That's what we do. But our focus, as the bridge, is not on the brain; it's on patients' behavior. Parents are not coming in to ask us, "Is there something wrong with my kid's brain?" They're coming to us to ask, "Why are they having these problems or what problems might they have in the future?"*
>
> —*Keith Owen Yeates, Ph.D.*

An effective feedback session allows the patient and family to develop a better understanding of their diagnoses, cognitive scores, and expected prognosis. Through the feedback session or sessions, neuropsychologists have the opportunity to meet patients and their families where they are, within their unique set of cognitive, emotional, and cultural contexts, and help them to understand what it all means.

> *We put it all together. One doctor tells them to take medication for their abnormal EEG, and the school tells them that their child is having trouble, and another doctor tells them that their child has ADHD, but no one puts this together for them. One of the things I consistently get feedback from patients and even from some physicians, is when they tell me, "I learned more today than I have learned after talking to doctor after doctor over the past 10 years." Because what do neuropsychologists do? They spend time with their patients.*
>
> —*Michael Westerveld, Ph.D.*

Neuropsychologists use feedback sessions to help patients understand their particular neurocognitive syndromes in the larger context of their real-world environments, in an empathic and therapeutic manner. This process offers the patient and his or her family hope and empowers them as advocates. How do neuropsychologists achieve this? The answers are like the feedback sessions themselves—varied and complex.

FEEDBACK'S IMPACT ON HEALTH, HOPE, AND PATIENT ADVOCACY

At its core, the feedback session is an opportunity to explain in detail not only our assessment results, but also more generally the neurological conditions that patients bring to our offices. Remembering the purpose of our feedback sessions can help us provide the information that patients and families most need to hear. Many have never had the opportunity to sit with a doctor and hear in detail what happened to their brain following their stroke, or what the expected course following a traumatic brain injury looks like. Feedback sessions are an opportunity to provide a basic understanding of the patient's condition. This understanding then becomes a framework on which we can hang our assessment results.

> *When people come to us, it's because they are hurt somehow. The hope is that they will get a better understanding of what is wrong with them and what they can do about it. Our feedback is one of the few opportunities to convey to the people who have been evaluated what the meaning of the assessment is for them, what the recommendations are and how they fit with their brain functioning.*
> —*Robert M. Bilder, Ph.D.*

Once educated, patients can become collaborators in the feedback process, which then helps them better understand the impact or clinical meaning of our findings.

REFRAMING HOW PATIENTS VIEW THEIR CONDITIONS

The feedback session is an opportunity to assist patients and their families in changing the way they view themselves and "the problem." In fact,

> *Feedback sessions are often as much about debunking myths as they are about sharing information.*
> —*Gail Grodzinsky, Ph.D.*

Along these lines, feedback can be seen as a process of framing and reframing the narratives that patients and their families bring to the assessment so as to help them "own" the clinical formulation.

> *Everyone comes in with a narrative about why his or her child is having trouble. And there are often multiple perspectives. The mother might have one narrative. The father another. The school often has another narrative. So you want to listen to these impressions. Sometimes you can say, "You were really right. You know your child." Other times you have to say, "You know, I can see why it looks this way, but in fact...."*
> —*Deborah Waber, Ph.D.*

FEEDBACK AS A PSYCHOTHERAPEUTIC MOMENT

Feedback is the primary treatment that we offer as neuropsychologists. Almost universally, the clinicians we interviewed noted that feedback, when done correctly, can be an intervention in itself, and that our primary training as clinical psychologists is critical to that therapeutic success. Part of that training allows us to sit with patients as they grieve, and even invite that grieving process. Neuropsychologists also use therapeutic skills when gauging the emotional temperature in a room, and in pitching our discussion of issues to what we feel is emotionally relevant at that moment. Many patients' underlying concerns involve questions like, "Am I crazy?" or "Am I getting dementia?" Approaching those questions directly—and quickly, can be an essential therapeutic process.

> *They are anxious, so I start with a little psychotherapy. Relieve the anxiety. I don't start with a bunch of numbers they aren't ready to hear. If the neuropsychologist does not provide information that the patient wanted in the first place, then it's a waste of time for both the clinician and the patient.*
>
> —*Marc Norman, Ph.D.*

Feedback in neuropsychology is not just individually therapeutic, but is fundamentally a systems intervention that can include the family, school, and/or workplace. Neuropsychologists rely heavily on their clinical training in understanding the nature of systems and ways their interventions have an impact on multiple layers of the system. At times, the focus of the session shifts from the immediate needs of the identified patient to those of their spouse or parents.

> *I feel that neuropsychology is the best marriage therapy, no ifs, ands, or buts. A patient's wife now understands what the miscommunication is, sometimes after years of misunderstanding.*
>
> —*Cheryl Weinstein, Ph.D.*

For some patient populations, feedback messages are pitched as a "cure" for the primary clinical problem. For example, feedback sessions can be an opportunity to give people with somatoform disorders an exculpatory out; in the hands of a skillful clinician, these sessions can help move patients toward seeing psychotherapy as a helpful tool, rather than as a dismissing message from another medical professional who surely must think they are "crazy." Guiding a patient to a place where they can see psychotherapy as a concretely helpful option is a delicate therapeutic intervention in itself. Some neuropsychologists will take multiple sessions to provide feedback, particularly with somatizing patients. In these instances, feedback can look very much like brief psychotherapy.

Beginning with the initial interview, we are entering patients' and families' lives. The degree to which we utilize therapeutic skills may be a significant contributor to how well we are able to gather information and data, and how well our formulations and recommendations will be acted upon.

HELPING PATIENTS AND FAMILIES BECOME BETTER ADVOCATES

When patients and their family members understand their neuropsychological conditions, an opportunity arises for them to become more effective advocates. One poignant, and common, example of this is the family with a middle-school child who is still not reading. Parents who did not realize their child had dyslexia, and spent years being reassured by school professions that their child just needed "the gift of time," will frequently become tearful in feedback sessions. Once they understand the diagnosis and available treatment, parents can become successful advocates for their children: because they finally know what to ask for, and how to ask.

An effective feedback session explains how psychological and neurological factors interact to produce the clinical presentation. Understanding these interactions empowers family members as they navigate school or other community systems. This knowledge can also guide family members of adult patients to understand what will be helpful, and not helpful, in their own interactions with the patient. John J. Randolph puts it beautifully, "I want my patients to walk out my door with ideas to pursue. I don't want them walking out without ideas."

> It's my belief that we should try to change something about the family's and the child's lives with our exams. If we don't, our exams aren't really helping all that much. We change their lives by giving them new information, and helping them change the perspective they take when thinking about their child and their child's situation. We also change their lives by helping them to become empowered advocates. If we just give them good information and they walk out the door and nothing happens, then we didn't do our job. So it is our goal to do something dramatic with the assessment and the feedback session, so when they walk out the door, they will be inspired, empowered, and have access to new resources. So they can do something that can change their child's life.
>
> —Mark Mahone, Ph.D.

ON GIVING PERMISSION

In reflecting on the question "What is feedback?" one unifying principle that emerged was that of giving permission. Neuropsychologists offer patients and their families permission to expose their vulnerabilities and to ask questions they may have been too afraid to ask, as well as to cry, grieve, and hope.

Permission to expose vulnerabilities

Adult patients often come to our office afraid that our testing results will confirm their greatest fears. Family members might hold back important information for fear of negative evaluation or criticism. Our current medical system (and reimbursement model) often requires physicians to see patients over increasingly shorter periods of time. Because of these restrictions, even the best medical doctors can be perceived by patients as rushed and therefore impatient or inaccessible; a context that makes it challenging for patients to expose their vulnerabilities. In contrast, neuropsychologists have the opportunity to spend a considerable amount of time with patients and their families. This allows us to create an environment that feels safe, non-evaluative, and importantly, not rushed. This environment essentially gives permission to patients or family members to share things they may have spent considerable effort hiding.

> My clinical training has taught me that I am stronger than any one patient's psychopathology. Parents may feel ashamed to tell you some things. If you open the door, they can tell you, "In my worst moments, I did this...." If you don't create a holding environment, that can't happen.
>
> —Janine Stasior, Ph.D.

Permission to ask questions

Many clinicians have had the experience of finishing a feedback session, only to have the patient or a child's parent timidly ask if it is "okay" if they ask one more question. For example, one of us once had a parent ask, "I heard that if you have children too close together in time that it will cause problems for the second child. Is that why Johnny has all of these problems?" In this case, the child was 10 years old, and the mother had been carrying this unnecessary guilt all this time, because she was too afraid to ask the question—and to discover whether it really was "her fault." The time she spent with the clinician, the trust she built in that relationship, allowed her to take that risk.

Permission to cry

Neuropsychologists frequently see patients and families who have lived through life-threatening medical events or have struggled for years with developmental disabilities. In the assessment process, many patients and their families work very hard to keep themselves emotionally together. They may be in the habit of presenting themselves as emotionally nonreactive to protect the patient, other family members, and friends. Our office may be one of the few environments that give patients and their families permission to express their distress at the events that brought them to us.

> *When we talk about difficult topics, parents grab the Kleenex box. Their job is to be there for this kid, they aren't supposed to let down their guard in front of their kid or other people. The parents are my client, too, though, and I specifically make a place for them to let down their guard.*
>
> —*Molly Warner, Ph.D.*

> *Sometimes it's a matter of just letting them cry in my office because they haven't had a safe place (away from the child they don't want to scare) to do that yet. Human connection is, I think, a powerful thing.*
>
> —*Hillary Shurtleff, Ph.D.*

Permission to grieve

Many clinicians emphasized that by providing emotional space within the feedback session, they allow parents, spouses, and other caregivers to process their grief.

> *Giving parents space and your presence to grieve provides so much hope, because it validates their feelings, validates them as people. Providing that presence, and not just rushing through data was hard for me when I first started. Now I joke sometimes that I make mothers cry for a living!*
>
> —*Hillary Shurtleff, Ph.D.*

> *What parents need from the professional neuropsychologist is a segue—a way to step into the nature of their loss. I'll often say, "Let's just notice that this is*

sad...." Once a professional does this, it's almost like granting parental permission to express feelings.

—*Paul Kaufmann, JD, Ph.D.*

Permission for family members to consider their own needs

Depending on the family dynamics and presenting problems, feedback sessions can become a moment to offer permission for spouses to consider their own needs, and the needs of their children. For example, feedback with families of individual's with Alzheimer disease often focuses on education and support of family members. The dementing individual may feel physically sound and have no awareness of their cognitive deficits, and is therefore not identifying themselves as "the patient." The family, in contrast, is experiencing distress and seeking assistance. In these situations, the family system can be seen as the primary focus of therapeutic intervention.

Permission to hope

Of course, the most important gift we can offer patients and their families is hope and proportion.

> *You asked how I give people hope. Sometimes it's a matter of educating them about the details. When dealing with acute medical issues, people seem to find so much support by defining what they're dealing with. Sometimes it's a matter of just listening and validating their observations and feelings. Sometimes it's a matter of listening to their concerns and addressing them. Sometimes it's a matter of helping to reframe issues. Sometimes it involves getting them involved with support groups or other parents or resources online, or educating them about how strengths can be used to compensate for weaknesses. Usually it's a combination of things. There are just so many ways to help people hope.*
>
> —*Hillary Shurtleff, Ph.D.*

> *In our clinic we want parents to leave with a sense of optimism. We really try to focus on what their child is good at. The school may never see it. They may not have learned these things in school, but it is important to honor it.*
>
> —*Deborah Waber, Ph.D.*

LEARNING TO GIVE FEEDBACK

Historically, many senior and even mid-career neuropsychologists were not explicitly taught how to give feedback. Some clinicians shared with us that they were *discouraged* from offering feedback during the early portion of their careers. Consequently, a large number of clinicians have learned how to give effective feedback "on the job." That raises the question: How have we learned to do this extraordinary task well? Remarkably, as the field of neuropsychology's focus has shifted to the identification of ever more complex cognitive processes, with hundreds of books available describing sophisticated assessment methods and neuropsychological syndromes, there has been almost no parallel literature describing techniques for communicating this information to patients and other professionals.

The exception to the silence in this area is Tad Gorske and Steven Smith's contribution, *Collaborative Therapeutic Neuropsychological Assessment* (Gorske & Smith, 2009). Their work is based on a movement in the psychological assessment field to include patients in an active process of collaboration, from the beginning of the assessment. The movement was initiated in the 1970s by Constance Fischer. In response to a perception of psychological assessment as objectifying, she introduced the concept of "collaborative individualized assessment." (Fischer, 2000). Similarly, "therapeutic assessment" is a parallel technique of evaluation and feedback that views the entire process of assessment as a therapeutic intervention (Finn, 2007). These methods involve dialogue and collaboration, as well as deviating from standardized procedures throughout the assessment process in order to arrive at a more holistic understanding of the patient's inner world. While such changes in test procedure may not fit with some clinicians' practices, the underlying theories can be applied to improve the quality of feedback by integrating the patient into the assessment process and thereby including their perspective during the feedback session.

Despite the increasing complexity of the field and high level of skill required, many neuropsychologists do not learn to provide feedback through formal instruction. Graduate programs universally require coursework with names like "Assessment Methods," but few programs offer courses dedicated to the complex task of giving feedback. Trainees typically learn feedback techniques through informal methods. Medicine's classic model of "See one; do one; teach one" predominates. Interns might sit in on a mentor's feedback sessions and eventually be supervised when giving their own feedback. Some internship and postdoctoral fellowship programs are beginning to place a more active emphasis on this skill and its development, but these programs appear to be a relative minority in the field to date.

Even without a formalized curriculum, learning through observation allows for its own educational process. Many neuropsychologists shared how they picked up their mentors' metaphors and stories that made complex concepts accessible to patients and their family members. Metaphors, stories, and "pearls" that are effective in communicating results and explaining complex concepts simply and effectively are handed down from mentor to student and shared amongst colleagues informally. That said, how neuropsychologists give feedback often has much to do with their personality, as well as their family and regional background.

> *I speak plainly. The bottom line here is that if I weren't a neuropsychologist, I would probably be a farmer. So the feedback discussions are plain and simple. We didn't learn any of this in our training. This is from our own parents and experience.*
>
> —*Michael McCrea, Ph.D.*

This is an important point. Trainees do not leave fellowships providing feedback exactly like their supervisors do. In fact, some neuropsychologists whom we interviewed shared that they learned what *not* to do by observing their supervisors, especially when watching a style of feedback they did not wish to pursue. Some pearls and communication styles fit with their personalities and their eventual clinical setting, others do not; some pearls stick with them, and others will be left behind.

In addition to picking up feedback strategies during their training in neuropsychology, clinicians also tell us that over the course of their careers, they have reached back to their primary psychotherapy training to "figure out" how to provide feedback. Most have also hit upon their own metaphors and ways of providing feedback through trial and error. When patients and family members begin to nod, those metaphors are filed away as a useful approach to a given population. If the patients' eyes glaze over, that particular analogy might not be used again.

This book presents a unique opportunity. We have conducted in-depth interviews with over 85 neuropsychologists from all over the country: training directors, members of tertiary medical teams, private practitioners. We are offering readers the ability to be a "fly on the wall" as these seasoned neuropsychologists provide feedback to patients across the lifespan, with a wide variety of neurological and developmental conditions. Like receiving the best feedback training from 85 different mentors, we have gathered the most compelling, accessible ways of explaining complex neuropsychological concepts from a broad variety of practitioners.

Some of these pearls will fit with your personality and the needs of your clinical population and practice setting. Others will not. Trainees will enter a candy store filled with clinical opportunities. More seasoned clinicians will read through and spot pearls they immediately recognize will help them communicate more effectively. On a personal note, we have found that as we gathered pearls, we "took them for a test drive" in our own clinical practices. Just as with a new car: we drove at first cautiously, maybe a little awkwardly. But with a few repetitions, many of the pearls became our own. The neuropsychologists who contributed to this book have generously offered up their compelling feedback messages, strategies, metaphors, and stories that effectively synthesize complex information. Go ahead and try them out your own practice. Deborah Waber notes that during feedbacks her team's goal is to paint a portrait of the child, in all their complexities. With that in mind, consider this book a deluxe set of paints.

REFERENCES

Finn SE. *In Our Client's Shoes: Theory and Technique of Therapeutic Assessment*. Mahwah, NJ: Lawrence Erlbaum Associates; 2007.

Fischer CT. Collaborative, individualized assessment. *J Pers Assess*. Feb 2000;74(1):2–14.

Gorske T, Smith S. *Collaborative Therapeutic Neuropsychological Assessment*. New York: Springer; 2009.

Pegg, P., et al. The impact of patient-centered information on patients' treatment satisfaction and outcomes in traumatic brain injury research. *Rehabil Psychol*. 2005;50(4):366–374.

2   Why Some Feedback Sticks

THE QUESTION OF what makes communication effective has been addressed in the literature of every branch of social science. Neuropsychologists are typically familiar with one or more psychotherapeutic theories that address not just content (what to say), but delivery of therapeutic messages (how to say it). Motivational interviewing is one such communication technique that has been recommended as helpful in delivering neuropsychological feedback (Gorske & Smith, 2009). However, neuropsychologists may be less familiar with communication theories and techniques that arise from other social science fields.

Brothers Chip and Dan Heath, one a professor of organizational behavior at Stanford Business School and the other an educator, bring a novel perspective to the topic of effective communication in their book, *Made to Stick: Why Some Ideas Survive and Others Die* (Heath & Heath, 2008). They draw from folklore, marketing literature, and more traditional communication theory to address the question: Why do some ideas, like the urban myth about kidney thieves, rapidly spread and persist despite being untrue, while other, scientifically sound, ideas are hardly noticed? Their focus on how to effectively communicate intrinsically complex or boring ideas that are outside a listener's typical framework of understanding makes their work particularly useful for neuropsychologists.

The Heaths point out that when an idea sticks, "we understand it. We remember it, and we can retell it later. And if we believe it's true, it might change our behavior permanently" (Heath & Heath, 2009:4). This is exactly the goal of neuropsychological feedback. How can we make the communication of complex assessment results and neuropsychological processes compelling and memorable? Although the goal of this book is not to offer communication theory, and suggest that readers construct their own feedback metaphors (we freely give these away in later chapters), we feel a discussion of the Heaths' compelling ideas provides a helpful framework for understanding the effectiveness of the many feedback strategies clinicians shared with us.

Before providing specific methods for communicating information in a compelling manner, the Heaths provide a tangible example of how to make complex information accessible to a targeted audience. They share the story of the Center for Science in the Public Interest (CSPI), a nonprofit agency tasked with explaining nutrition to the general public. CSPI's goal was to address the high amount of saturated fat in popcorn made with coconut oil. This movie theater popcorn included 37 grams of fat (almost twice the daily recommended allowance of 20 grams). Understanding that there was nothing compelling about the concept of "saturated fat," the CSPI's campaign eschewed the typical graph or table presentation, and instead provided something much more tangible. During a press conference, they announced that a medium-sized bag of popcorn contained as much fat as a "bacon and egg breakfast, Big Mac and fries for lunch, and a steak dinner with all the trimmings combined!" All of that food was laid out on a table for the cameras. The general public became so turned off to movie popcorn that sales dramatically declined, and theaters were ultimately forced to stop using coconut oil. A clear message for neuropsychologists from this example is that even ideas that are innately scientifically dry can be "made to stick."

One of the key messages in *Made to Stick* is that ideas do not need to be "dumbed down" in order to make them compelling. However, the Heath brothers also point out that as scientists, attorneys, or accountants, we are accustomed to speaking and thinking in the particular language of our professions. The assumptions and jargon that we work with every day become invisible to us. When we communicate to "the general public" we lose sight of the jargon we use and forget that others have never heard of our basic assumptions. Our messages are not compelling: not because they lack merit, but because our audience cannot access them. The clever dissertation of psychologist Elizabeth Newton was shared to demonstrate this concept (Newton, 1990).

Dr. Newton sorted groups of subjects to either be "tappers" or "listeners." Tappers were asked to tap out the rhythm of 25 common songs, like "Happy Birthday" or "Edelweiss." Listeners were to guess what song was being tapped. The tappers were asked to predict whether their listeners would successfully guess the songs. Even though the task was actually very difficult, tappers could hear the song in their head as they tapped out the rhythm. Consequently, it seemed to them that discerning the song when hearing the rhythm would be quite easy for the listener as well. They predicted that listeners would accurately recognize their song 50% of the time (or one out of every two songs). In reality, only three of the 120 songs tapped were accurately guessed in the entire experiment.

The Heaths comment that the job of a tapper is particularly difficult because *they* know the song, and cannot help hearing the tune as they tap. It was very difficult for the tappers to understand that their listener did not have the same advantage. To them it was the most obvious thing in the world, and they seemed equally oblivious to their listener's dilemma. Rather than assuming the problem was with them, they assumed that there was something wrong with their listeners. The Heaths label this basic problem of communication in our highly specialized culture: "The Curse of Knowledge," noting that, "once we know something, we find it hard to imagine what it's like to not know it." Dr. Newton commented in her text, "The tapper and observer subjects were so embedded in their own imaginations—so caught up in the richness of the melodies they were 'hearing'—that they could not recognize how impoverished the stimulus was from the perspective of the listener" (Newton, 2009:44).

While not described in the Heaths' book, but of particular interest to neuropsychologists who supervise students, Dr. Newton's experiment went on to include "observers" who had neither the experience of being "tappers" nor of being "listeners." These observers were told the songs, and then asked to watch the interactions between the tappers and listeners. Like the tappers, they also incorrectly predicted that guessing the songs would be relatively easy for the listeners. This demonstrates that even from a distance, it is difficult to empathize with the perspective of a listener who does not have the advantage of hearing the tune in their head. Once the knowledge of the song is present, taking the perspective of those who have not heard the song is a very difficult task, even from the distance of being an observer.

The take-home message from this research is clear for neuropsychologists. We are tasked with communicating complex assessment results with patients while the "music" of our knowledge of neuroscience, neuroanatomy, and psychological principles is clearly playing in our heads. It might be easy to recognize this mismatch in communication as we watch trainees plow through a recitation of standard scores and drop terms like "diaschesis" to patients and their families, but it may be more challenging to spot the problem in ourselves after years of practice. In some ways, neuropsychologists might be even more likely, given the nature of our patient's cognitive impairment, than the tappers in Elizabeth Newton's study to attribute the lack of understanding of our message to a lack of cognitive capacity in our listeners; they do not understand our results because they cannot understand, not because we have failed to make the results accessible. But of course, this is a temptation we must avoid if we wish to ensure that our messages are *heard*. The second phase of the experiment also highlights that even supervisors can fail to recognize the source of a patient's difficulty in understanding our findings.

THE SIX PRINCIPLES FOR MAKING AN IDEA "STICK"

In analyzing compelling ideas, the Heaths propose six principles that make an idea "sticky." They suggest that ideas that are simple, unexpected, concrete, come from a credible source, trigger emotions, and include stories tend to stick. As we interviewed neuropsychologists about their stories, metaphors, and communication strategies, we recognized many of these principles at work. To illustrate the principles, we will present outstanding exemplars from the "pearls," some of which you will also see in Part II of the book.

Principle 1: Simplicity

Midway through a neuropsychologist's long, complex explanation of standard scores and expected developmental trajectories, family members might start to get a glazed-over look in their eyes. A parent's thought bubble might begin to devolve into worry about the ultimate punch line: "Does John have ADHD? Will he have to go to a special ed class? My father-in-law is so anti-medication. Will he become like that zombie kid down the block?" Or the child or spouse of an elderly patient may begin to focus on their own worries about a possible dementia diagnosis and its associated number of challenging, emotionally draining decisions.

Many of the neuropsychologists we interviewed emphasized that patients and family members can become anxious in feedback sessions when overloaded with too much information. To avoid this situation, many intentionally present families with only two or three points, especially when giving bad news.

> *I know what those points are before I go in. I tell them within the first 10 minutes, and then spend the rest of the hour dealing with it.*
>
> —E. Mark Mahone, Ph.D.

Simplifying the feedback message—bringing it to a basic core idea—allows the message to gain traction and guides the actions of patients and family members. This principle of simplicity is illustrated in *Made to Stick* by the military concept of "commander's intent." This is a very useful concept for neuropsychologists, particularly when educating families to go out and advocate for their children in Individual Education Plan (IEP) meetings or with state agencies.

Commander's intent is based on the principle that no military plan survives contact with the enemy. Commanders could spend endless time creating highly detailed plans for combat, but these could easily go awry based on unforeseen circumstances. Making the commander's intent clear to those in the chain of command allows soldiers to improvise as necessary to meet the goal. The commander's intent might be, "By the end of the day, we want to take that hill." How the hill is taken is up to the soldiers on the ground. Two questions are often asked to ensure that officers understand the commander's intent: "If we do nothing else during tomorrow's mission, we must _____"; and "The single most important thing we must do tomorrow is _____." Similarly, neuropsychologists might ask themselves prior to a feedback session, "If I do nothing else during this feedback session, I want to communicate the fact that Sam _____." Or the goal might be to have their patients leave with a clear plan of action: "If we accomplish nothing else during the IEP next week, we want to ensure that _____."

Principle 2: Unexpectedness

Before you can get a patient or family member to understand and remember what you have to tell them, you have to get their attention. Prior coming to you, many patients and family members have sat in chairs across from other clinicians' desks: neurologists, primary care physicians, perhaps even school principals or special education directors. Is your message disappearing amongst multiple other encounters with professionals?

The Heaths' second principle for creating sticky messages is unexpectedness. This is consistent with the well-established neuroscience principle that humans orient towards novelty. Ideas that are unexpected will be better remembered because we pay more attention to them in the first place. What will the family take home from the feedback session? Most likely it will be the part of your message that grabs their attention by being delivered in a novel, unexpected manner.

Yana Suchy shared a wonderful analogy for explaining the prognosis for deficits following a stroke that perfectly captures this element of unexpectedness. She likens normal brain function to 10 men carrying a log, and the effect of stroke as some of those men becoming injured. In an acute hospital setting, with beeping monitors, and residents discussing cerebral blood flows and blockages, this analogy is startling.

> o *"You have 10 men carrying a heavy log. A couple of them get injured and leave. Then you have eight men left carrying the log. At first it's hard, but eventually they get stronger and stronger and then they can carry the log. But sometimes, you get a situation in which eight of the ten men get injured and leave. Then you only have two men carrying the log. Then it takes a long time. They will eventually get stronger. As long as there are some men there, you can eventually improve. But for the duration, even when the men get as strong as they can, the log is carried more slowly. There are only two men carrying that log. And of course, in the situation in which all the men get injured—there are no men left to carry the log. In those situations, function is not going to return."*
>
> —*Yana Suchy, Ph.D.*

When family members get on the phone with relatives to explain what they know about Dad's condition, you can bet they will talk about that log.

What if your child's neuropsychologist takes off his shoe and begins waving it in the air during the feedback session? Unexpected. Michael Santa Maria shared this method for explaining a dry concept to parents. How do you help a child recall instructions when their verbal memory is relatively weak? Many parents (or professionals at IEP meetings) do not have a clear idea of what "help him rely on his visual memory" actually means. It's one of those abstract concepts that elicits nods, but is then quickly forgotten.

o *"Your son's visual memory is much better than his memory for words. So if you tell him to go upstairs and get his shoes, he may come down a half hour later without them. So, do this"* (Mike takes off his shoe and waves it in the air) *"Hey! Go upstairs, get your shoe!"*

The doctor actually took off his shoe during our feedback session! This is startling enough that the family will not forget the technique.

Principle 3: Concreteness

The Heaths point out that language is abstract, but life is not. We have several hours worth of test data to communicate. Our feedback is more likely to stick if we can explain, concretely, what those scores mean for a patient's everyday life. Mark Barisa's method of explaining why it is not safe for a patient to drive is an excellent example of this principle of concreteness. When families minimize risks ("Oh, Dad only drives to the grocery store and back"), rather than present abstract concepts like "complex attention" or "visuoperceptual abilities," Barisa reminds families how inherently demanding driving is.

o *"Think about all that goes into making a left hand turn across traffic. You're judging your own speed, and your own reaction time. At the same time, you are judging the other car's speed. A lot goes into it."*

In this manner, families are given a concrete explanation of how Dad's thinking changes will effect his driving. Yes, he might be able to operate the car, but now they have a concrete explanation for why he cannot operate it *safely*.

Principle 4: Credibility

Establishing credibility can often be the first step in helping families take home the complex messages we are presenting. Taking a cue from his mentor, Jane Bernstein, Mark Mahone brings people into his office and sits them facing his diplomas.

> *They will find it easier to accept me as an expert. I am telling them strategies for helping their child that maybe their mother in law has said is a terrible thing to do (e.g., considering psychotropic medications for their child). I am asking them to trust my recommendations, and this makes it easier.*

A key element in an idea that sticks is a trusted source. For example, the Heath brothers point out that urban myths almost always begin with, "I have a friend whose cousin … " or "A study at [*fill in the prestigious university*] found.… " In the healthcare field, trust has traditionally been established by one's credentials as a doctor. However, the current climate of competing experts and information overload may sometimes erode this traditional trust in clinicians.

Consider a common parenting experience. Every parent has at some point, had to get an overtired, howling infant to sleep, while trying to juggle the conflicting advice of experts: "Let the baby cry, it's a natural process of settling down. If you don't let them cry it out, they will be sleep-deprived and unable to self-soothe." Or, alternatively, "Don't let the baby cry. The tears are a natural mechanism for alerting parents to a real need. If you let them cry it out, you are disturbing the natural attachment process." This conflict amongst credible professionals leaves parents wondering, regardless of the method they choose, "Am I hurting my baby?" Many parents give up on the experts and call their own parents for advice. For sleep-deprived, stressed new parents, it is hard to forgive the experts for not getting together, coming up with a single, clear, answer, and sticking to it.

This competition of expert opinions is common in our information culture and may lead to an overall distrust of experts, scientific facts and data. CNN and other networks have created a visual format for this type of competition with boxes, where competing experts have their own sections on the screen. There may be five or more boxes filled with arguing professionals on a single display. When expert opinions conflict, or an overload of medical information becomes too much, patients and families may revert to looking to their immediate communities, or perceived immediate communities for advice. This is why some families come in to consulting rooms with web-based printouts, feeling that personal testimonials of various treatments from people with children "just like theirs" have greater weight than abstract scientific studies.

Under the right circumstances, clinicians can take advantage of this principle and establish credibility by sharing their own personal stories or those of other patients. This also helps to convey their understanding of the emotional layers the family is experiencing. For example, Hillary Shurtleff gives children an example of a prior patient to model how another adolescent was able to successfully use psychotherapy.

> o *You know, I just saw a 17-year-old who had the same surgery you had about a year and a half ago (temporal lobe resection). She had gotten really depressed and she went to see a psychotherapist. It was really helpful to her. She was having some trouble with her parents because they were so over-protective. The therapist helped her figure out how to be more independent, how to talk to her parents about this.*

The teenager hearing this message may not have trusted the neuropsychologist as a credible source, but hearing about another teenager who has gone through the same medical experience may well convince her.

Similarly, when encouraging patients who are hearing-compromised to wear their hearing aids, Muriel Lezak takes her own hearing aids out and puts them on the table in front of the patients. She increases the credibility of her message by establishing herself as an individual who also has hearing loss.

> o *I make no bones about it. I say, "If you need them, you need them. You're not just making your own life miserable, but you're creating a terrific burden on your family. Your wife is suffering and only you can help."*

Principle 5: Emotions

"Belief counts for a lot, but belief isn't enough. For people to take action, they have to care." The Heaths point out that even if an idea is credible, it may not be effective unless emotions are engaged. The idea that emotions contribute to an idea's "stickiness" is consistent with the well-established literature on the enhancing effects of emotions on memory, at all stages of the memory process. As neuropsychologists well know, emotional stimuli are prioritized in situations of competing stimuli (Kensinger, 2004). Emotional arousal and either negative or positive valence also enhance encoding, and information that is emotionally arousing is better consolidated. In contrast, neutral information tends to decay over time (LaBar & Phelps, 1998).

Michael McCrea demonstrates this principle when he talks to patients about driving. The abstract concept that one *might* get into an accident is not as compelling as the emotional loss of one's legacy:

> o *"I know in this country driving is our ticket to independence. But you don't want your legacy to be 'the guy who ran over the kid on the bicycle.' I remember about three years ago an older person lost control of their car at O'Hare. Drove right through the front of the airport. Into the building. And my first gut reaction is, he might have worked 50 years as a schoolteacher, he has 27 grandkids. But he's going to die as the guy who ran into O'Hare Airport. You don't want to be the guy who ran over the kid on the bicycle."*

Principle 6: Stories

Stories transform patients and families from passive listeners to active imaginers. As neuropsychologists, we know that when we imagine, the same neurocognitive systems in the brain are activated, just as if the experience were actually occurring in "real life." This is most famously illustrated by the elegant study of the imaginings of Italian stroke patients whose neurocognitive systems were not working in "real life." Patients with left-sided neglect, and who were all very familiar with the Piazza del Duomo, were asked to describe the famous landmark. Remarkably, depending on where they were asked to imagine standing in the square, they would neglect to describe the buildings and landmarks to their left. Asked to imagine standing on the opposite side of the square, they would describe what they had just previously left out (buildings that had previously been on the left), but were now on the right side of the imagined space (Bisiach & Luzzatti, 1978).

Imagination's activating effect on neurocognitive and neuromotor brain systems is also illustrated by the phenomenon of mental practice improving real-life skills. This has been demonstrated in music and in sports (Driskell, Copper, & Moran, 1994). When subjects imagine themselves practicing musical instruments or their short games in golf, they improve their actual abilities. More recently, mental practice has been used to improve surgical skills in residents (Arora et al., 2011).

When we tell a story, we invite patients and families to enter into an active rather than a passive feedback moment. Rather than receiving information, we provide a visceral experience of the point we wish to make. For example, when Joe Ricker discusses the prognosis of recently severely brain-damaged individuals, he will often share the story of a teenager he worked with whose clinical picture was initially so hopeless that he was almost placed in a nursing home. When told in all of its detail (see pearl in Chapter 10: Traumatic Brain Injury) the punchline of the story, "Everyone thought he would be in a nursing home, now he's a senior in college," helps families to identify and access two important threads: 1) there *is* hope for amazing gains, well beyond what we predicted; and 2) *but* he still has deficits. Storytelling allows patients and families to directly imagine this nuanced message in a manner that is impossible when the clinician is relying solely on statistical information to share the likely outcome.

Similarly, Jim Irby shares stories about other patients with similar difficulties, when working with brain-injured patients suffering from an impaired awareness of their deficits.

> o *"I've worked with a lot of guys your age who have had the same kind of problems. Let me tell you about that (here is where you shift off of them to someone else who is like them). Now you may or may not fit this. But let's talk about others who have had this type of injury and see whether it might fit you. Here's how it goes...."*

> —Jim Irby, Ph.D.

In this way, patients are able to let down their end of the rope in what is typically a constant *"I'm* fine; *you're* sick" tug of war and "try on" an explanation for their current set of frustrations. The story allows them to drop their defenses because it is not about them.

As neuropsychologists, we have the music of our knowledge of neuroscience, neuroanatomy, and psychological principles clearly playing in our heads. While this knowledge is why our patients come to see us, it can also act as a barrier to their leaving with a full understanding of their assessment findings. It is our responsibility to actively devise ways to allow our patients to directly hear that music in the richest, most compelling fashion possible—so our feedback sticks.

REFERENCES

Arora S, et al. Mental practice enhances surgical technical skills: a randomized controlled study. *Ann Surg.* Feb 2011;253(2):265–270.

Bisiach E, Luzzatti C. Unilateral neglect of representational space. *Cortex.* 1978;14(1): 129–133.

Gorske T, Smith S. *Collaborative Therapeutic Neuropsychological Assessment.* New York: Springer; 2009:58–60.

Heath C, Heath D. *Made to Stick: Why Some Ideas Survive and Others Die.* New York: Random House; 2008.

Heath C, Heath D. *Made to Stick: Why Some Ideas Survive and Others Die.* New York: Random House; 2007.

Driskell JE, Copper C, Moran A. Does mental practice enhance performance? *J Appl Psychol.* 1994;79(4):481–492.

Kensinger EA. Remembering emotional experiences: the contribution of valence and arousal. *Rev Neurosci.* 2004;15:241–251.

LaBar KS, Phelps EA. Arousal-mediated memory consolidation: role of the medial temporal lobe in humans. *Psychol Sci.* 1998;9:490–493.

NewtonE. *The rocky road from actions to intentions* [unpublished doctoral dissertation]. Stanford, CA: Stanford University; 1990.

Ibid., p. 44.

3 Feedback Protocols and Theoretical Considerations

DURING ONE OF our initial interviews for this book, Gail Grodzinsky made a point that was subsequently emphasized by many others: "there is no protocol for giving feedback." That said, as our interviews progressed, we began to recognize familiar patterns, which eventually sharpened into several recognizable feedback strategies. This is not to suggest that all clinicians follow the same sequence in a feedback session, or even that they share the same beliefs about *what* patients should be told (e.g., see "Using the 'A word' [Alzheimer disease]" in Chapter 6). Furthermore, a single clinician may utilize multiple strategies depending on patient and family characteristics. However, many common strategies were seen across clinicians regardless of their clinical setting or patient population. This chapter presents these strategies. Like the rest of this book, it is our intention to provide multiple examples of approaches that work for neuropsychologists, rather than suggesting a single "correct" way to structure the sessions.

FEEDBACK BEGINS AT THE CLINICAL INTERVIEW

When we asked clinicians to describe the flow of their feedback sessions, we were repeatedly reminded that the feedback session starts with the first patient contact. While some suggested that feedback started as early as the first contact with the office, most emphasized the intake session, because it allows neuropsychologists to set the stage to effectively share their findings. Some clinicians begin to provide concrete feedback during the intake itself. More commonly, however, this time is seen as an opportunity to build trust, enlist patients and family members as active collaborators, and foreshadow information that will likely be covered during the formal feedback session. The initial evaluation is also typically used to assist families and patients in framing their questions for the assessment and managing their expectations. At the same time, it allows the examiner to explore potential defenses that patients and families may have to the primary diagnoses being considered. This groundwork leads to more collaborative and useful feedback sessions.

> *Feedback is driven by the initial interview and mediated by assessment. If the history is done well, then during the feedback session 90 percent of your work is done. You know what the family's concerns were, what their theories were, the theories of the school, and so on. You can clarify and articulate for the family the referral questions you know you will be able to answer. Those questions and issues provide the fundamental place where you begin feedback.*
>
> —Karen Wills, Ph.D.

For many clinicians, a significant focus of the initial interview is to simultaneously track and gather information to both make the diagnosis and facilitate feedback. At times the same information might be used for both purposes. Other information is elicited specifically to support the feedback process. For example, many neuropsychologists shared that they are deliberate in their use of the clinical interview as a mechanism to gather information about the biases family members might hold, with the purpose of later using this information to strategically encourage them to accept and even embrace findings that they might otherwise deny or reject. An excellent example of this process is the strategy of asking all family members their theories of why their child cannot read. The answers provide input that is useful for diagnosis, and also forewarns the clinicians if Dad or Grandma feels Charlie is just "lazy." Should the assessment prove them wrong (and it typically does!) understanding their biases prior to the start of the feedback session allows clinicians to address the "laziness issue" as part of their overall feedback strategy. It also encourages buy-in from family members who might otherwise feel that their theory, "He's lazy," was never considered or assessed. For another example, clinicians might solicit information about the patient's fears in order to inform them how to directly relieve those reservations or how to best break the news gently and effectively.

The process of concurrently attending to diagnostic and feedback issues during the initial clinical interview is reminiscent of a seasoned therapist's ability to listen to their patient, while simultaneously entering into a reverie about therapeutic resonances and strategies. In this manner, the clinician is already considering the topics they will cover, the obstacles they want to work around, and even the specific language or metaphors they will employ to most effectively convey their message.

> *The interview is so important for planning your feedback—figuring out what these people already know. What their level of sophistication is, what kind of questions they are asking me. All of that helps me to frame what I'm going to talk about in the feedback session; for example, what kind of vocabulary I use.*
>
> *—Katrina Boyer, Psy.D.*

> *What we do a lot even as early as the interview, is begin to make some judgments based on the interactions with the family, about what they can tolerate and what metaphors or what examples to use. So if the person is academically inclined, I might plan on bringing more written material for them to read or some website references. If they seem less academically focused, if I look at their questionnaires and there are spelling or grammatical errors, I might be more likely to bring the old brain model to the feedback.*
>
> *—Michael Joschko, Ph.D.*

ESTABLISHING TRUST

Establishing trust during the initial interview leads directly to improved collaboration during the assessment itself as well as a shared understanding and construction of the ultimate message during the feedback session. Part of establishing trust involves reassuring patients about what the tests may uncover. Patients can be very anxious during both the assessment and the feedback session, which makes them less likely to effectively process the feedback message.

> *Some patients feel like a terrible secret will be revealed, or they will be made to feel stupid. The message I want to convey is that we need THEM to do our job well. This helps them more comfortably engage in the testing process. They are already in a collaborative mindset, and therefore they are less concerned about what the testing will reveal. .*
>
> *—Gordon Chelune, Ph.D.*

THE IMPORTANCE OF EMPATHY

Closely related to building trust, is the important role of empathy.

> *Early on I realized that empathy is the key to giving feedback. Can you imagine what it would be like to be parents, sitting there hearing from someone they didn't know well that their child was cognitively impaired? There is an art and a science to neuropsychology. That's how I try to live my professional life. Originally I wanted to be a therapist, but found neuropsychology during graduate school. I have continued to maintain that humanistic part—whatever impulses led me to psychology in the first place. When it comes to feedback, I can't rely on much to distance me from patients' pain and my compassion comes through. That seems to ease patients' pain.*
>
> —*Joel Morgan, Ph.D.*

One aspect of empathy is curiosity and a willingness to ask questions, rather than assume information about patients. This is important during the initial consultation, when interview data is collected, and during feedback sessions, when clinicians must determine how clinical formulations and recommendations are being digested by patients and families.

> *I get so mad at students when they put words in patients' mouths. One time a patient's wife said, "I've been married for 25 years." And my student said, "Oh that's great, such a strong relationship." I gave that student a look to kill and said to the patient's wife, "Is that how you feel?" (Because I had a feeling it wasn't.) "No," she said, "My husband is so mean to me."*
>
> —*Roberta F. White, Ph.D.*

At times the psychological issues of family members will get in the way of their ability to "hear" feedback. This can be related to guilt, if for example, a parent perceives that they are responsible for the child's problem. On other occasions, parents may be irritable or angry with the child who has a longstanding issue, like ADHD, but whom they perceive as a "lazy kid who just isn't trying." Trainees often fall into the trap of perceiving defensive parents as being difficult, rather than as people in pain. Sometimes even more-experienced clinicians can be overwhelmed by the emotions of a family member and how they express themselves during clinical interactions. In both of these instances, this can set up an unproductive dynamic in the feedback session.

> *I tell trainees, "You need to respect every parent who walks in the door. Each parent has different tools. You need to figure out what. What do you know about this person's life that puts you in a position to judge that they are dealing with this situation inadequately? One, what are they dealing with? Two, who are they? What tools has anyone ever given them in their life to deal with a child who has spina bifida? The number one resource a child has is their parent. And as the clinician, one of the most important things you can do is listen to and support the parent."*
>
> —*Karen Wills, Ph.D.*

When clinicians are able to understand the dynamics of the larger system, or "holding environment" in a Winnicotian sense, these issues can be explicitly or implicitly addressed in feedback. They can also help build the clinician's empathy, which in turn will increase the level of trust and rapport with the patient and family.

Linda Vincent takes another approach to enhance her ability to empathize with families. She meditates prior to the initial and feedback sessions in order to increase her connection with a patient's experience. She notes that the improved sense of empathy has been one of the most rewarding experiences in her professional career.

> *Meditating prior to an interview or feedback session assists me in being open to the unknown person coming in my door. I am better able to be present with that individual, as opposed to thinking about all of the things I have to do or the phone ringing in the other room. I am trying to focus on their situation. I might for example meditate on how hard it is for them to come in to see me. Or what it would be like to come in with whatever their story is and tell it to a total stranger. It's really developing my own theory of mind. Prior to feedback sessions, I try to imagine as best I can what it would be like to come in and to hear the news that I am about to give. Dementia, or some other diagnosis—maybe the patient doesn't want to hear. I try to think about that and to be respectful. I reflect on being empathic and gentle in the way that I get to my findings, taking care not to get ahead of the patient. This process of meditative preparation has been really helpful for me. I carry patients in a different way inside me, as compared to those I have seen in the past. I remember them better. Since I have been doing this, I have been getting a lot more "thank you's." People will call and ask if they can see me again—it's much more personal and connected. I am the one who is different—not the patients.*

For some trainees and clinicians, empathy can come almost too easily. Several neuropsychologists talked to us about the difficulty in balancing their professional role while working with the many emotionally challenging components that patients and their families bring to the table. These conversations highlighted the need to balance empathy and a professional emotional detachment to most effectively do our jobs.

> *I try really hard, in feedbacks that I know will be difficult, to disconnect myself emotionally. I try to focus on what my job is. I come back to the referral question. I care about these kids and sometimes I find myself really wanting to help some of these families—you know, they pull you in for whatever reason. They have a lot of emotion tied into this situation, and I want to be respectful of that. I want to empathize with that, but the way I can be the most helpful is to focus on what my job is. They're depending on me to do my job and to do it well.*

> *What can I do, what are the limits of what I can provide? What can't I do? And I try to be precise with that, and not worry about things that I can't provide for this family. That's an important lesson for fellows to learn. A lot of the time when a fellow is overwhelmed in a case, just focusing them in on what is their job in this case can help. We're not involved in issues of custody, and so forth. Let's focus on what question is being asked of us—that is our question. There are a whole slew of other*

things that are important, but they are not our problem, so let it go (send them to someone who can help with that problem, but let it go). This helps in detaching just enough in order to do our job. In psychology we have a tendency to want to take on the whole child and the whole family and while having knowledge about all of that, seeing how your patient fits into that context, it's not your problem to deal with the whole thing. (It helps to work in a medical center where resources are available to refer families for support.)

—*Katrina Boyer, Ph.D.*

This is not a recommendation to remain distant and unconcerned about the distress our patients bring to us. Rather, it is a recognition that we, as providers, can sometimes best help our patients and their families by remaining focused on the details that we can effectively help change. Of course, helping families connect with hospital and community resources that provide wraparound services is also an important component of caretaking that can further support our interventions while allowing us to focus on our piece of the puzzle.

FRAMING REFERRAL QUESTIONS

Many neuropsychologists emphasized the need to clarify our patients' specific questions and goals for the assessment.

My goal during the clinical interview is to take parents' concerns and worries, and help transform them into specific questions that can be answered by the assessment process. I will revisit those specific questions during the feedback session, using the language the parents brought in. I find that the best pearls during feedback sessions are often from the parents' own mouths.

—*Janine Stasior, Ph.D.*

Some of the goals brought in by patients and their families might not be achievable in the context of the assessment. For example, when working with the geriatric population, we might hear, "We want to find out how Mom can get her memory back." In these instances, the initial interview becomes a venue to manage the expectations for the assessment process. Other goals are important to patients and their families, but may not have been a central part of the initial referral question, such as "I want to find out if Mom is okay to snowbird in Florida independently this year." Clinicians can carefully note those goals, so they can be directly answered during the feedback session.

UNDERSTANDING PRECONCEPTIONS

The initial interview also provides an opportunity to understand patients' and families' pre-established ideas.

If you know how a parent or patient thinks about the problem, then you can frame the feedback in those terms, and bring them to a different understanding. For example, in the initial interview, you could say, "So, Dad, how do you feel about why Johnny isn't doing well in school?" If he answers, "He just doesn't want to do well," then in the feedback session, I am sure to say, "Yes, motivation may be a part of this, but he also has...."

—Gerry Taylor, Ph.D.

Some clinicians include a question on the intake form, such as, "What do you think is the IQ of Dad_____, Mom_____, Child_____?" If, for example, the parents estimate their own IQs to be "High Average" and their child's to be "Average," the clinician knows that the parents understand that something is amiss with the child's IQ. Being aware of this prior to walking into the feedback session makes a difference in terms of how information about the child's IQ can be presented. Indeed, as noted above, in addition to gathering information to assist in the differential diagnostic formulation, we heard over and over again about how many questions posed during the diagnostic interview can be simultaneously designed to help facilitate the feedback session. For example:

> *I find that many parents are apprehensive about having their child diagnosed with ADHD. Some of them are in complete denial, even though their child has been literally bouncing off the wall and/or pretending to swim across the testing table while working with me. In order to help parents appreciate the collaborative nature of the assessment process, and to help me get them to accept an ADHD diagnosis, I tend to be very blunt about the question during the interview; I put it on the table for them to help me figure out the answer. I usually say something like, "Given the history you have shared so far, and some of my interactions with Johnny, one of the primary differential diagnoses I need to consider is ADHD. Let's go through it together. Tell me why you think Johnny might have ADHD, and why you think he does not." Once I get this information, I can usually help the parents correct their misperceptions, and see more of the child that I have been observing. By doing it during the interview, though, I get one more advantage. I can say to them, "I am sharing my initial thoughts with you and thinking out loud on purpose. We still have another day of testing" (or, on those occasions when I haven't met the kid yet, "I haven't even met Johnny, so obviously I'm not diagnosing him"). "I want you to spend some time considering what we have talked about. If you find yourself agreeing with me, and start recognizing features you had overlooked before, share this with me at our next appointment so I can build those examples into the report. On the other hand, if you really think I am missing an important point or an alternative explanation for these impressions, then let me know and we will explore the topic together some more when we meet again."*
>
> *—Kira Armstrong, Ph.D.*

Mark Mahone describes a similar strategy:

> *I start giving feedback and shaping the intervention for the family and child from the moment of first contact. I set up the initial interviews with them in a way that, in addition to gathering information, I am also getting a feel for where they are in their belief system, and where they are in terms of their understanding of their child's conditions and sequelae, and of course their misconceptions about things.*

A lot of what I do is work to change misconceptions right off the bat. I work to lay the foundation for the feedback that I am ultimately going to give. For example, the parents might say during the initial interview, "My child is really bright" (and I know he is really lower functioning). I might say, "What does he do that makes you say that?" If the parents respond with a misconception, "He's definitely bright because he can recite entire episodes of TV shows by rote memory," I will immediately correct that assumption, spending some time talking about what intelligence really is. This is to set the stage to ultimately tell them that their child is low functioning in the feedback session. I will start, in the first meeting with the family, to challenge many of their beliefs.

This kind of approach offers the parent and/or patient a sense of involvement in the diagnostic process; they are working *with* you to find an answer. It also provides the clinician information that is needed to help the patient work around their fears, avoidance, or denial. Similarly, clinical observations about the patient and the family can further direct *how* feedback is ultimately presented:

I watch the interaction of patients and their parents closely, with an eye for sources of conflict and whether a family member is wedded to a particular expectation. How traumatized are they? Are the tears near the surface, or not so near the surface?

—Brenda Spiegler, Ph.D.

PROTOCOLS FOR THE FEEDBACK SESSION

While there is no formally endorsed protocol for feedback sessions, there are stages that many clinicians utilize. These include re-establishing rapport, reorienting the patient to the assessment process and goals, providing a summary of testing findings, and directing the patient and family towards community resources and intervention options.

Reorienting the patient and family

Just as it is important to set the stage during the initial interview, how one initiates the feedback session helps to create a productive environment for the patient or family to receive our findings. For example, reminding patients and their families that this is a collaborative process can help them re-engage and renew the relationship established during the initial interview. Steven Guy opens his session by reminding parents: "I prefer this to be a conversation. You are the expert on your child. I want you to jump in, agree, disagree. Tell me what you think. Please ask questions as we go along."

Although some directly discuss their collaborative approach with patients and families, other neuropsychologists use their clinical skills to effectively invite family members into the dialogue. For example, they may make a few statements and then stop and wait, literally allowing time for family members to consider the findings and then enter into an exchange of ideas. Neuropsychologists likewise use their clinical skills to monitor the effectiveness of their communications, checking in with patients and family members to ensure, "Am I getting them where they need to be?"

> *My job is <u>not to say</u> what the brilliant neuropsychologist thinks. It's an opportunity to clarify what the patient thinks, and what their plans are going forward—and how those plans incorporate the information we learned during the assessment.*
>
> —*Robert M. Bilder, Ph.D.*

Reviewing the family's goals for treatment and your alignment with them can also build on this process. For example, Michael Westerveld opens his feedback session by explaining:

> *"What I want to do is make sure that we are on the same page. You had questions when you came in here, and we talked about those questions during our first meeting. I approached the assessment based on what I understood those questions were. And so to start the feedback, I want to make sure that I understood properly. If I didn't, before we get too far talking about the data, I can shift my focus towards what you were here to learn." I will then restate my understanding of the referral questions the family came in with.*
>
> *I also orient parents to the feedback process by stating, "I understand that there are multiple levels here: One of course is 'How's my child doing after their accident [or surgery]?'" A lot of times parents also have the desire to understand the "why" a little more; what's happening in the brain that is causing these changes. And then the "What next?" So I might say something like, "My understanding is that you wanted to know why Charlie is having trouble with his friends. And as part of that question, there is a diagnostic question that your physician had: does he have autism, or is something else going on? Depending on the answer to that question, you want to know how to help him, and where do we go from here?"*

Similarly, Brenda Spiegler initiates the conversation by stating:

> *"Tell me again what your concerns are." This lets them know that this is going to be a dialogue. It also gives me another chance to direct my comments to their concerns. Also, when a family member is there at the feedback session, but not [the] interview, this gives me an opportunity to hear his or her perspective.*

As described in Chapter 1, feedback sessions are not just about providing a patient and their family with a diagnosis. It is an opportunity to empower the patient and family by providing them with information, resources, and next steps. Barbara Schrock opens with this premise when working with stroke and TBI patients, noting:

> *"The purpose of our meeting today is for me to be a resource to you. I feel knowledge and information is control. The more information you have, the better choices and decisions you can make in your life. It doesn't do me any good to have this information about you—you need to have it." I also typically add, "I want to make sure I address any questions and concerns you might have. You may have figured out that it is hard to give a straight answer about anything when it comes to recovery. You may have heard conflicting answers. After 30 years, I may not know all the answers, but I bet I have heard all of the questions."*

When working with children with identified genetic or congenital conditions, the etiology is already clear. In these instances, families are specifically participating in a neuropsychological assessment to help them develop and follow meaningful clinical interventions. Given this premise, Andrew Zabel begins feedback sessions by asking parents to restate their goals for their child:

> *"In terms of life skill functioning and independence, what do you most worry about? And what are the things that would bring the most quality of life improvement?"*

Gathering more information and solidifying formulations

While feedback sessions are an opportunity to provide information, they are also a chance to gather additional information from patients or family members and to test diagnostic conclusions. In many child assessments, one parent might have been available during the clinical interview, but both parents attend the feedback session. An opportunity arises to gather more history and hear from family members who have not yet expressed their view of the problem. Similarly, in many geriatric cases, multiple family members will come to hear the results. The primary caregiving sister might have brought Mom initially and provided the history, but the concerned brother from out of town might provide a very different picture of his understanding of their mother's needs during the feedback session.

Feedback sessions are also often used to gather additional information from the patients themselves, which can further extend the assessment process. For example, many neuropsychologists routinely ask how patients felt they did on the tests.

> o *"So, how did it go for you? I'm sure after you left here you had a lot of thoughts, some happy, some not, about the experience. How do you feel it went?" Their answer tells a lot about their level of insight. Some people felt it went great, when they bombed; some are convinced it didn't go well when their profile is completely normal.*
> —*Michael McCrea, Ph.D.*

> *Feedback, just like the initial interview, is this open-ended thing, where you try to get the patient to tell you what the issues are. If they think they have brain damage and you think they don't, and you do the feedback correctly, it is very likely they will tell you why.*
> —*Roberta F. White, Ph.D.*

This process not only informs the neuropsychologist further about how to deliver their findings, it rebuilds rapport, which is an essential component to helping the patient process his or her test results. When giving feedback directly to children, Hillary Shurtleff emphasizes that:

> *Rapport is essential. And it's hard to establish that without showing sincere interest in the child (which is easy for me as I really enjoy children). For kids, I typically first find out where they are, "What was hard or easy for you?"*

Starting with a compliment was commonly reported, no matter what age the patient is. "Wow! That was a lot of testing, huh?! You did a great job getting through it all. I was really impressed." Or, "Johnny was really motivated for the testing. He clearly tried his best."

Being flexible

Following a protocol is an important tool to help clinicians organize the emotionally charged information we have to share with patients. However, being flexible can be just as important.

> *I have a plan, but I go with the flow. I start by saying, "First of all, I haven't seen you guys for a month. Any new news? Anything that's happening that you want to start by telling me, before you hear about the results of the assessment?" Then I move on to, "Okay, when we talked a month ago, what I understood to be your main concerns were, 'xyz.' Have I got that right?" Or, "As you had a chance to think about it, was there anything else that I need to be thinking about so I make sure to address your concerns?" In doing this I remind them that we already have a relationship; I already know these secrets, maybe things that feel shameful to them about their family and child. And it's going to be okay. I will rearticulate that in a way that feels solution focused; they present it as problem focused, and I will restate it as solution focused. This comes straight out of doing therapy. We are not just going to sit here and slam your kid. Now they are hearing the problem a second time, in the context of results.*
>
> —*Karen Wills, Ph.D.*

Leading with the bottom line

Following introductory comments, clinicians have a choice to make: lead with the bottom line, "You were right to be concerned, Jane does have significant reading problems," or begin more broadly, either with data or general descriptions of brain function and dysfunction. Many clinicians emphasized their belief that it is important to introduce your conclusions early during the feedback session.

> *I will very quickly say to parents, "I am going to tell you the bottom line." I used to give parents much more detail, but I found that they could not absorb the information. It detracts from our reframing; parents are interested in the recommendations. That's why they came.*
>
> —*Deborah Waber, Ph.D.*

> *I cut right to the chase in the beginning, where I used to build to a crescendo.*
>
> —*Steven Guy, Ph.D.*

> *Every evaluation should start with a question and end with an answer. For example, is this person likely to do well after a temporal lobectomy? Do they have Alzheimers? I start with, "This is why we saw you." And then I tell them right away what the answer is. I then continue with as much supporting evidence as they appear to want to hear.*
>
> —*Christopher Grote, Ph.D.*

Leading with the bottom line can be particularly helpful in situations where you are in a position to share good news: "I know you have been anxious about your memory, but I want to start off today by telling you that your memory is entirely average for someone your age." Patients can breathe a sign of relief, and are better able to listen to details once their anxiety has been allayed. Even when the news is difficult, leading with the bottom line can allow patients and their families to listen more attentively to details later in the session, rather than focusing on whether the dreaded diagnosis will ultimately be made. Of course, this approach is equally effective with pediatric populations.

SHARING THE DATA

While many clinicians highlighted the advantages of sharing the diagnosis first, many others prefer to lead with the testing data, describing strengths and weaknesses in each of the cognitive domains, often illustrating with performance on a particular test.

> *I typically walk them through the test results themselves, highlighting areas where their performance was normal or abnormal. I go domain by domain.*
>
> —*Michael McCrea, Ph.D.*

Greg Lamberty also begins feedback sessions with the test data.

> *Over the years, from a consumer standpoint, I felt that that was a good thing to do. Patients think, "I spent all that time doing those tests, so what the heck were they all about?" The level of detail is dictated by the patient or family's ability to understand. With bright folks, I spend a fair amount of time talking about tests. It's either overwhelming or quite helpful. Even when overwhelming, I get the feeling that people feel glad that I took the time to explain specific results. In pediatric cases, it's almost always the case that the families are ready and willing to hear more.*

Sharing the specific data is also a mechanism to help patients and their families understand and accept your findings:

> *You need to provide the patient with information on the examination, what they did and how they did. I recommend that you start with the strengths. I developed a worksheet that I still use. I can use this worksheet to say, "Look, here are all your strengths," and I'll point to their average or a few high average or superior scores. "Look how good you are on this, this, and that." I actually show them the worksheet so they can see concretely they have some strengths. When they come in for an examination they are devastated. They are keenly aware of what is not working well. They generalize—"I am stupid." "This sheet very concretely demonstrates my point: you are not stupid."*
>
> —*Muriel D. Lezak, Ph.D.*

As discussed in Chapter 1, other clinicians rarely discuss specific test results, and avoid detailed descriptions of numbers. Clinicians who take a more middle ground may discuss a subset of scores, or highlight a patient's performance by domain, but spend considerably less time discussing actual scores or taking a test-by-test approach to review the results.

Beginning with broad concepts

Some clinicians begin by educating patients and family members about broad concepts of brain functioning, typically with the help of brain models, before addressing specific issues relating to the patient. These neuropsychologists emphasize the common findings in the patient's disorder (e.g., TBI or CVA) and ask the patient, "Which of these symptoms do you feel you are experiencing?" The neuropsychologist then uses this as a direct segue to explain the patient's specific testing results.

> I feel the first task in the feedback session is to provide the survivor and family with a conceptual framework upon which they can then hang the details and the information I will give them later. After explaining what neuropsychology is, I let them know I will be giving them my little 10-minute lecture on how the brain works. This is absolutely canned I can do it in my sleep. After teaching patients about brain systems, I collaborate with them in predicting what their own deficits might be, given the location of their lesion....
>
> When there is a stroke, or an Arteriovenous Malformation (AVM) we look at particular areas affected for the patient. "So now that you know all of this, what can we expect?" (Patients now collaborate with me. For example, I might say, "You had an AVM. Here is where it was. Now what would YOU expect?") This method normalizes the deficits. It all makes sense. You lead patients to those conclusions, so they don't feel it's awful or demeaning. You are treating them like a person who can think. A collaborator. "Now we can start talking about what happened to you, and what your strengths and weakness are. And what recovery looks like."
>
> —Barbara Schrock, Ph.D.

Christopher Nicholls also begins by providing a primer on brain function and explaining specific neurocognitive syndromes to patient's families. For example, when providing feedback about a child with dyslexia, he will bring up a PowerPoint presentation on his desktop computer screen. He then provides a 10-minute "Intro to Neuropsychology" lesson, including concepts of posterior vs. anterior, left vs. right, and then brain differences in dyslexic and non-dyslexic readers. He introduces the child's scores in the context of this background information.

> I then return, verbatim, to the questions gathered from the family during the initial interview, "Here was one of your questions. This is what I think.... Here's the next one.... This is what I think." If they are nodding, and agreeing, "That's it! You really nailed it," I will then say something like, "Doctors have to use labels to talk about things. Here's the label." When they have been nodding, and you say, "and that's what we call ADD, or dyslexia" ... they hear it better. If you have woven a story, describing behavior and symptoms, they have bought into it and agree with you, they are ready to hear what to do.

Cheryl Weinstein refers to the practice of educating patients about brain function as "Neuropsychology 101," and presents the information over the course of a handful of feedback meetings. She introduces the idea to her patients by "inoculating them" against the desire to avoid the topic.

> *"I'm going to teach you about neuropsychology. It's a course that I would love to take. But you might not want to take it, because you want to hide all these problems. You don't want anybody to know. But life is easier if other people know."*

"I hope I am wrong"

Sometimes, we have to share diagnostic or prognostic impressions that can be difficult to hear, especially when families are not quite ready for the information. These situations most often arise when a patient's injury or illness leads to a change in their expected lifetime trajectory (e.g., an acquired brain injury, dementia, or other progressive disorder), or when a child's developmental limitations require parents to change their expectations for the future of their son or daughter. Sharing this information is often done strategically and delicately. Many clinicians also very carefully and intentionally leave the door open for alternative expectations, such as preceding the information with an "I could be wrong" statement that, as James Irby points out, "leaves the door of hope open." John Beetar notes,

> *I believe as a person that you have to have hope. I think to myself, "I hope I'm wrong. They have dreams for their children. I hope that what I say is wrong. I hope one day they will come into my office and wave something in front of me that proves 'You were wrong!!'"*

To encourage a family's hope while still sharing the full constellation of possible outcomes, some clinicians overtly encourage the patients and family to hope we are wrong.

> *When working with pediatric traumatic brain injury, I was often faced with parents who had been told on numerous occasions that their child might never do this or that again. This left them emotionally crushed, but when the predictions were wrong, it also led them to distrust medical experts and the information they shared. One of my mentors (Kim Kerns) taught me an especially effective way to work around this situation. Even though I no longer see many children with TBI, I find it is still a helpful way to convey results that parents might otherwise find overwhelming or too negative to take in. I say to parents, "It's my job to educate you about the best- and worst-case scenarios. I'm going to tell you what we can hope for, but also what long-term limitations your child might have. Your job is to hope for the best. With any luck you will come back to me in the future and say, 'You were wrong!' and I truly hope that will happen." This allows the parents to hear what I have to share without having to fully accept my prognostic impressions. More importantly, they don't feel like I am forcing them to believe in something they aren't ready to accept. In this manner I can discuss all of the worst-case scenarios without losing them or our professional relationship in the process.*
> —Kira Armstrong, Ph.D.

MULTIPLE FEEDBACK SESSIONS

For neuropsychologists who work on hospital services, or in research programs in which patients will be expected to return many times, feedback sessions are often seen as an opportunity to build a relationship. In these situations, neuropsychological services are viewed more as a longitudinal process than as a single consultation. Consequently, there tends to be less concern about comprehensively providing scores and cognitive information during the first feedback session with families. Instead the focus might be on gaining their trust, developing immediate treatment plans, and helping families see the neuropsychologist as a resource over the course of a long treatment relationship.

> *I don't want to just give families a one-hit wonder. As a neuropsychologist I try to take them from stage to stage. To do that in the feedback session, I am making a connection, not just explaining results. The therapist in me has to come out. For example, I won't just go into a meeting when a family is in denial and try to force something on them that they are not ready to hear. If you do the legwork up front, there are no surprises in these meetings.—James Brad Hale, Ph.D.*

Similarly, many of the neuropsychologists who work in hospital settings talked about the extended relationships they build with families through their follow-up evaluations and subsequent feedback sessions.

> *I work with the family and the child throughout the child's development—not as a one-shot assessment. I integrate information from many other professionals for the family, and will often act as a resource when the family needs to maneuver [through] other medical and educational systems. To communicate this I tell patients' families, "I work like your family practice doc, when it comes to services that are in support of your child's brain."*
>
> *—E. Mark Mahone*

He adds that if you have a child with a brain disorder, it is likely to be a lifelong condition.

> *We set them up at the beginning with an expectation—"We will be taking care of your child for the duration." I don't feel pressured to answer every question right away, because I set up our work together as something we can do over a period of a few months or a few years or a lifetime. More often than not, I see them a few times. I help them with the intervention that we recommend afterwards, and then I see them back in a few years. In the interim, I ask them to get a hold of me and tell me how things are going. I might do things for them that takes me 10 minutes, but can have a major impact on the child's life. Most of the questions in between our assessments I can answer in five minutes, but they really help the family.*

Even when clinicians work in outpatient settings, there are occasions when one feedback session is not enough to provide the patient or family with the information they need. Some neuropsychologists work around this situation by holding a second, more remote feedback session or "check-in session" where patients and family members provide feedback to the neuropsychologist about what recommendations have worked, and what have not. A course correction with additional recommendations can then be devised.

Finally, feedback sessions can also be an instrumental mechanism to ensure that families follow through on referrals to other professionals. Karen Wills frequently makes appointments for her patients while they are sitting in her office, because she knows that many of them will not be able to do it independently. She will then schedule a follow-up feedback session to integrate the outcomes of those appointments with her treatment plan:

> *"Here's the timing of the next training session through the learning disabilities advocacy group for you to find out about your rights. I want you to be there. Let's call them up and get you registered. Then, come on back, I will see you in a month or two, and we can talk again about our plan for education intervention in the school."*

4   How Is Feedback Presented?

THIS CHAPTER IS not about the words that are used during a feedback session. It is about how the conversation is set up—and just as important, how the words are delivered. Who is invited to listen to the feedback message? How long will the conversation last? Does it take place in person, over the phone, via e-mail? What social pragmatics are employed or emphasized, such as tone of voice and degree of authority invoked? In the course of our interviews, we found that the "how" of feedback is often as interesting, if not more so, as the "why" and the "what." Depending on the patient population, geographic location, clinical setting, and predilections of the neuropsychologist, the physical characteristics and social pragmatics of feedback sessions can be systematically varied to achieve clinical goals. Our intention with this chapter, as with the rest of the book, is not to describe what should be done, but to present a variety of strategies, and their rationales, that work well for different clinicians.

THE PHYSICAL SETTING

The typical physical setting of a feedback session is in the neuropsychologist's office, with patients and family members on the other side of a consultation desk. However, neuropsychologists who work in inpatient settings are equally likely to give feedback at a patient's bedside. In these situations, clinicians generally attempt to create as much privacy as the situation allows. For example, they may determine when the patient's roommate will be out of the room for his or her own treatment or testing, and choose that time to deliver the patient's results. While most clinicians indicated they prefer in-person feedback, feedback can also be delivered outside of the classic consultation room or office model.

Hallway conversations

Some of the most important information may be conveyed *after* the diagnostic interview, assessment or feedback session occurs. For example, while escorting the family back to the waiting room (following the diagnostic interview), Gordon Chelune will often slow his pace so that he is walking next to a family member. This allows him or her to ask questions they felt they could not in front of the patient. He might also repeat information, or rephrase it in a way that applies specifically to their caregiving concerns. This emphasizes that he understands the impact of the patient's needs on their own emotional adjustment. Similarly, Michael Santa Maria often takes an opportunity to pull aside a patient's spouse or adult child after the formal feedback session, particularly when giving feedback to an individual with anosognosia, who cannot appreciate his or her limitations. This allows him to reinforce certain concepts such as, "It's too early for your husband to return to work; he doesn't want to lose his reputation."

Feedback by telephone

Many neuropsychologists who work in rural settings or tertiary care centers offer their patients feedback sessions via telephone, particularly when patients have to travel great distances to be tested and want to avoid an extra trip. Although many clinicians appreciate the benefits of this process, they also lament how challenging it can be to "read" how well patients are processing the information over the phone. For example, Jennifer Janusz emphasizes,

> *I never feel fully satisfied. Unless they are actively engaged, responding to what I'm saying and asking questions, I can't tell if they are confused or understand what I'm saying. I feel like I am giving only the basics and, for me it feels very awkward because I don't know what kind of information the parent is going away with.*

Interestingly, neuropsychologists' frustration with phone feedback sessions speaks to the natural feedback loop between clinicians and patients during an in-person session. When attempting to describe complex neurocognitive findings to patients, most clinicians are constantly looking to validate that their patient has understood the message. In person, we rely on body posture and facial expression, but we lose this feedback loop over the phone. Instead, we are left with the awkward mechanism of repeatedly asking, "Do you understand?" or "Does this make sense?" Relying on body posture and facial expression is a more natural, and probably more accurate, way to check in.

Some clinicians are in the early stages of investigating the use of Skype and other more HIPPA compliant video-streaming technology to rebuild their access to patient body language and facial expressions as the patient and family hear the feedback. At this point in time, access to a computer with a camera, required to use Skype, can be difficult for some low socioeconomic patient populations. However, as the technology becomes more common, primary care physicians who work in rural settings might be able to support such services by providing access to video-conferencing-ready computers in their offices. This would allow their patients to communicate with specialists in distant locations regardless of their economic status.

Feedback through e-mail

E-mail can be a convenient method of communicating with patients: Telephone tag is circumvented, some individuals who tend to ramble are naturally encouraged to streamline their questions and comments through this medium, and a record of the communication is instantly created and easily accessible. In some instances, e-mail can be the primary means of communicating feedback, although more typically, it is being used as a mode of providing additional information following a more formal feedback session. Aaron Nelson, for example, shared that he frequently utilizes (encrypted) e-mail to provide feedback, particularly with the "worried well;" he typically communicates results by e-mail when the news is good and he has already had a chance to briefly discuss the results over the phone. When clinically appropriate, he sends the patient's report with an e-mail that includes a brief introduction, such as:

> *"Overall your exam looked fine. I know you have been concerned about your memory. What you are experiencing is what comes with normal aging. In my note I have some recommendations for how you might address that. I enjoyed participating in your care. Please feel free to call me if you have questions."*

This is sometimes the beginning of a give-and-take over a number of e-mail exchanges that can be continued whenever he or the patient has the time to sit down at the computer. This mechanism also provides the opportunity to provide further information to patients after a more formal feedback session has been completed. For example:

> If I see a patient, and a family member has additional questions after the feedback session, and if they have permission and everything is okay from a confidentiality perspective, I will say, "Can you please summarize that for me in an e-mail?" I am not shy about asking people to give the information in an e-mail as a way to receive it.
>
> —*Aaron Nelson, Ph.D.*

LENGTH OF FEEDBACK SESSIONS

In the tradition of psychotherapy, most of the neuropsychologists we interviewed schedule an hour for the feedback session. There is some variability, however; some clinicians report that they schedule the feedback time to meet the needs of the patients and caregivers in the context of the complexity of the findings. This may require relatively brief periods of 15 to 30 minutes. For particularly complex cases, clinicians may schedule for an hour, with enough room in their schedule to run for 90 minutes or even longer, depending on the number of questions that arise in the course of the feedback.

TIMING OF FEEDBACK SESSIONS

The neuropsychologists we spoke with shared a number of different strategies regarding the timing of feedback sessions, although these were driven as much by the circumstances of the patient as by the clinicians themselves. For example, when patients travel long distances for testing appointments, many neuropsychologists provide feedback at the end of the testing day. For patients and their families who are overwhelmed with appointments, a return trip for a separate feedback session can be a significant burden. Allowing them to receive the information on the same day can decrease at least one of the many encumbrances the family is facing.

On the other hand, other clinicians specifically avoid giving feedback after a day of testing, because they are concerned that the patient is too wiped out to be a receptive consumer of information at that point in time. These clinicians intentionally arrange for the patients to return on another day for feedback. Still other neuropsychologists prefer to hold feedback sessions on a subsequent appointment because they send their reports to patients first, and then invite them to return when they can go over the report together. Interestingly, when the patient receives the report is also a matter of significant variation among professionals, and is discussed further in Chapter 16.

In addition to determining when a feedback session should be completed in relationship to the actual testing session, some clinicians described taking care to consider the time of day. These individuals talked about intentionally booking appointments at the end of the day. This allows them to be more flexible with the amount of time they can offer the patient, commenting that if the session needs to last an hour and a half, holding it at the end of the day allows that to occur.

WHO ATTENDS THE FEEDBACK SESSION

Although the guest list for adult neuropsychologists typically includes the patient, when working with children or individuals with dementia, practitioners vary in their strategies about when to invite patients to attend the feedback session.

Considerations for the adult patient

When working with adult patients, some clinicians always include patients, regardless of their cognitive limitations. Many cite the importance of having family members be able to refer back to the conversation as a primary rationale: "Mom, when we were all in Dr. Smith's office, he said you can't drive." On the other hand, some neuropsychologists choose not to include the patient, based on how well they are likely to retain the information. For example, when a patient has mild cognitive impairment or early Alzheimer's, most clinicians will include them in the process. If the patient is more advanced in the dementia process and is unable to lay down new information, then some choose not to invite them.

> *There is no value added, because they won't recall the information. Additionally, because they typically lack insight and don't see themselves in the same way as the test describes, the feedback sessions become a source of agitation.*
>
> —*Julie Keaveney, Psy.D.*

Of course, clinical decisions must always be made in the context of ethical guidelines. Therefore, when an adult is not part of the session, all of the neuropsychologists we interviewed emphasized their practice of obtaining releases of information, during the intake or testing session, to allow family members to hear the feedback.

Considerations for the child or adolescent patient

There are varying strategies for inviting young patients to feedback sessions. For Paul Kaufmann, children are always present during the first part of the appointment. He begins with the whole family and ends with the whole family. At some point "in the middle," a staff person takes the child into another room, which allows the adults to discuss topics like school placement, IEP team meetings, referrals, etc. Other clinicians we spoke to do not include children in the feedback sessions, preferring to spend the entire session speaking frankly with their parents.

In many practices, teenagers are given the option of attending, while younger children are not. Some practices offer a primary feedback session for parents, and a second, shorter session to explain the information directly to children or teens. Hearing the information about the need to make changes in their study strategies or the presence of a previously unrecognized learning disability, directly from the neuropsychologist, might have significantly more impact than hearing the information only from their parents.

> *I provide feedback to all adolescents, because it's critical for them to know who they are and to understand that they are not their disability. On the other hand, they must "own" their disability so they can advocate for themselves. I usually meet with the parents alone, and several days later I will have a separate feedback with*

the adolescent. I often use a visual (a pre-designed graphic organizer) to explain their learning style and then guide/brainstorm with the youngster management strategies. Afterwards, I invite the parents to join us and have the child summarize three major points (which we have rehearsed). The parents' job is to listen; we set up these rules in advance.

—*Gail Grodzinsky, Ph.D.*

A less common way to offer children their own personal feedback session is through letters:

I often write a letter to the child explaining his or her test results in easy-to-understand language. I always take care to emphasize their strengths, and give them a positive take-home message. I generally present the letter to the parents first, allowing them to proof-read it and confirm that they are okay with the content. I then mail the letter directly to the child. This process includes the child in the feedback process and gives them a concrete message about themselves that they can keep and read over and over again.

—*Kira Armstrong, Ph.D.*

The more the merrier: when the feedback session involves more than the patient

Robert M. Bilder includes his trainee(s), the patient, and anyone else who they can bring, in the feedback session. He feels that anyone who is involved in the patients' social network—spouses, friends, parents—should attend.

The more the merrier. The richer the network of people hearing the information at the same time—the greater the likelihood of something good coming of it.

Christopher Nicholls asks himself, who are the psychological stakeholders in the family? For example, if a grandmother is very involved, or if the stepmother is closest to the child, they should be at the feedback session.

Occasionally we have big cattle show with everyone there. If a big stakeholder is not there I might say something like "Golly, I'm surprised that Grandmother is not here, I know she was really worried about Johnny." Sometimes I can address the situation by "playing Colombo," to gently point out the lack of the important stakeholder in the room.

Deborah Waber encourages school personnel to attend feedback sessions via speakerphone:

Sometimes when people get an independent evaluation for their children the school can be put off, especially if you send the family off to the school alone with your report. You can use the feedback session to mediate. The school is generally very appreciative to be included. Sometimes the school will make a suggestion and the parents might say, "Well, if it's not in your report we don't want to do it." But through this process you can acknowledge when their advice sounds right. This can be a great relief to the family, and the school feels validated.

THE USE OF PROPS, TECHNOLOGY, AND OTHER RESOURCES

Many neuropsychologists use props to facilitate the feedback process. One of the most common props is the brain model, which is used to orient patients to various parts of the brain as his or her findings are described. Michael Westerveld tells us that he always has a brain model labeled with major functions in his office. He might say to patients:

> *"When you look at the EEG report, and it says 'left temporal spikes,' that's this area of the brain, where that spark is interfering with normal processing." Because the area is clearly labeled "speech," the parents can make their own connections such as, "Oh! This is why Sam loses his place when he is talking."*

The idea is to make it real, and concrete for people. Similarly, bringing a brain model to an IEP meeting, and beginning the presentation of neuropsychological findings by orienting team members to the relevant regions involved in the child's learning issues is an effective way to move the conversation from a discussion of test scores, to a discussion of this child's struggle to learn well in their particular education setting, given their particular brain dysfunction.

Some neuropsychologists have been keeping up with the latest advances in technology and now pull up interactive brain map applications on their iPads during feedback sessions.

> *These applications allow clinicians and patients to rotate the brain with their finger, and easily view different "slices" and 3-D regions. The technology is dazzling, and can engage teenagers and younger adults in the feedback discussion in a way physical brain models or an abstract description cannot.*
>
> —*Joseph H. Ricker, Ph.D.*

When practicing in tertiary-care centers, many clinicians have easy access to the brain imaging system of the hospital. Dedicated monitors are in most clinical offices, and neuropsychologists can bring up an MRI scan showing the patient's particular pathology. Most describe this as an excellent technique for patients or family members who may lack insight into the seriousness of the cognitive changes. The moment when the neuropsychologist makes the concrete connection between the cognitive or emotional findings and the patient's scan can be a powerful way to make the results more "real" for everyone involved.

Some clinicians use their computers to share PowerPoint slides that explain key concepts, such as neuropathology in right-middle cerebral artery strokes, or typical recovery curves following mild brain injury. Other neuropsychologists give patients and families journal articles germane to the feedback.

> *I find that parents tend to be very appreciative when they are informed about current research and are given copies of relevant papers. They see that you recognize that there are things unknown about their child's condition, and you are rolling up your sleeves just like they are, to understand the condition. You are in the same boat.*
>
> —*E. Mark Mahone, Ph.D.*

Sometimes the reason for using a prop or resource is to help a patient or family understand the seriousness of their condition and the need to make difficult decisions. For example, Michael

Santa Maria shares copies of a newspaper story about an elderly, cognitively impaired gentleman who crashed his car. The article includes graphic, even grisly photos, which make it that much harder to deny the risks the patient or family may have been attempting to avoid in making the decision regarding the patient's ability to drive.

Of course, an indispensable object in feedback sessions is the box of Kleenex. We were fascinated with the attention paid by clinicians to its placement in the room. Many clinicians consider the moment where they hand the box to a patient or family members an empathetic permission to express emotions. Others groaned at the thought of handing a box to someone, feeling that the gesture is a signal to the tearful individual to stop crying, and thus a way of shutting down emotions in the room. Neuropsychologists in the latter camp made sure to always keep a box in easy reach of family members.

SOCIAL PRAGMATICS OF FEEDBACK

How something is said is often as important as the words that are used when communicating with patients and their families. Tone of voice, body posture, facial expressions, even one's clothing serve to communicate the message behind the spoken word. For example, the same words, "Let's go outside" might suggest enjoying the air together, or the beginning of a fight, depending on the nonverbal channels of communication. These complex messages are referred to as "social pragmatics" (see Russell, 2007, for a review). When delivering feedback, neuropsychologists might consciously or unconsciously use social pragmatics to improve how their message is received. While some clinicians simply use the pragmatics they are comfortable with in day-to-day life, or what they saw modeled by mentors, others intentionally regulate their use of pragmatics as a clinical tool: titrating their eye contact, choosing social greetings, and setting their tone of voice to achieve specific goals. Extending the picture of neuropsychologists' using a paint box of metaphors and stories during feedback (as introduced in Chapter 1), social pragmatics can be thought of as another tray in the paint box, or an additional level of communication strategies.

Greeting patients

Feedback sessions begin with the neuropsychologist walking out to the waiting room, or into the consultation room, and greeting the patient and family members. How this greeting occurs varies from clinician to clinician, and can be strategically varied to set the tone for the rest of the encounter. Often clinicians are meeting family members for the first time: a daughter who flew in from out of town to hear her mother's dementia diagnosis, or a father who could not make the initial interview. Just as with the diagnostic interview, the neuropsychologist's use of titles or first names sets the level of formality. Decisions are based on, among other things, the cultural background of the clinician and patient, as well as each participant's age.

In many geriatric practices, neuropsychologists use formal titles—"Dr. Smith"—even though they may not use their "doctor title" when working with younger adults. In the geriatric age cohort, and in many ethnic groups, the expectation is for the use of formal titles; the use of first names can confuse role expectations and be distracting. Many younger clinicians, particularly women, point out that if they do not introduce themselves as "Doctor," elderly patients will assume they are a nurse or secretary. In fact, it is not unusual to have an elderly patient exclaim a few minutes after sitting down in the consultation room, "Oh! You're the doctor!" In pediatric practices, clinicians often introduce themselves to children as "Dr. Smith," but invite parents to call them by their first name. "Hi Sammy, I'm Dr. Smith … [turns to parents with hand out]: Dan Smith, nice to meet you."

A neuropsychologist may choose to heighten the formality of the setting by using a title, such as during an independent medical evaluation, or if they feel that less formality would facilitate openness, they might use their first name in the same situation. The take-home message is that the use of the formal title sets a specific tone, and can be used by the clinician to "dial up" or "dial back" the formality of the encounter to achieve specific clinical aims.

Similarly, clinicians must decide whether to use formal titles when addressing patients: such as calling a patient "Mrs. Barnes." This might feel awkward and contrived if the patient is the same age as the clinician. On the other hand, if a neuropsychologist has just referred to himself as "Dr. Smith," it might feel awkward or condescending to call the patient "Nancy." Equity or a consistency in use of titles is a standard fallback for most practitioners. Particularly in geriatric populations, most clinicians communicate respect to patients by using their formal titles: Mrs. Smith, Mr. Thomas.

Sometimes test results will suggest that the patient is unlikely to remember your name, or even who you are. In those situations, a "reintroduction" is warranted at the opening of a feedback session, to avoid having the patient's attention consumed with trying to orient herself to who you are and why she is sitting in the room with you. Of course, if you make the wrong call, and she knows who you are, or if she has just been cued by her son [whispered voice, "Mom, this is Dr. Smith," as you are walking into the waiting room], a formal introduction, "Mrs. Jones, I'm Dr. Smith" might be taken as an insult, or a sign you do not recall meeting her. Many work around this by offering a simple smile, along with their hand and a brief pronouncement, "Dr. Smith." This quick reference to one's name might be followed by a casual reorientation to the situation disguised as pleasantries while walking into the office, "It was so nice meeting you last Tuesday. You were so patient with our memory testing—not everyone is!"

Many make a point of offering water or tea at the opening of the feedback session (or during other appointments with the patient). This sets a collaborative, friendly tone.

> *I like to offer chamomile tea, which is considered a healing tea in Latino culture. The tea signifies warmth, and that this is a healing place. I also have food such as breakfast bars, crackers. I see many low socioeconomic status patients and always offer a breakfast bar/snack as patients may not have been able to eat prior to the session. In order not to shame them, I might say, "We're having a morning meeting, you might have rushed here. Can I offer you something?"*
> —*Monica Rivera-Mindt, Ph.D.*

Even the use of a handshake may vary and can be strategically introduced or withheld by clinicians depending on the clinical context. For example, sometimes a clinician may forgo this gesture when testing indicated the patient is clearly anxious (and might be ashamed of sweaty palms), has obsessive-compulsive disorder (and might not want contact with clinician's germs), or meets criteria for an autistic spectrum disorder.

Eye contact

Clinically, we often evaluate how our patients use eye contact as a means to understand how successfully they engage in their world. It is equally important to remember that our own eye contact can impact the effectiveness of our feedback sessions. For example, Mark Barisa cautions not to speak only to family members when a patient is in the room.

> *This would make anyone feel diminished: "Hey! I'm sitting here!" Instead, I orient myself to the patient, knowing there are people with big ears sitting close by who will be taking it all in.*

This can be a challenging skill-set for trainees to master, especially when they are still learning how to juggle all of the information in a patient's file and how to best share those findings. Some supervisors tackle this conversation head-on with their trainees, reminding them to:

> *Make good eye contact! And don't look anxious. Offer some professionally appropriate conversation. Don't just jump right in. Be warm and interpersonal.*
> *—Erin D. Bigler, Ph.D.*

This advice is especially important, as it can be easy to forget social pleasantries until a clinician has developed a real confidence in their feedback skills. Young clinicians may find themselves rushing to share findings, and in the process may also increase the patient's anxiety level.

Tone of voice and word choice

The tone of voice one adopts during a feedback session is not just predicated on a clinician's background and personality, it also can be a strategic method of connecting. Modulating one's tone of voice is an effective strategy for dialing up or dialing back the level of formality and authority in the feedback session. It can be especially important when working with psychiatrically fragile patients. Bernice Marcopulos describes using a very soft voice, with lots of verbal qualifiers, when giving feedback to inpatient psychiatric patients.

> *I use lots of "this may not be right, what do you think?" I am trying not to smack head on into their paranoia. I frequently check in, too, asking, "does this make sense?" I want patients to see the assessment as positive. If they have a positive feeling they might try some of the suggestions. It's about baby steps.*

Gordon Chelune describes his tone as "folksy" when working with most patients. He likewise maintains a soft voice, and leans forward in his chair, towards the patients. He specifically avoids using jargon. However, when working with some high-functioning, high-powered patients (such as a retired lawyer or CEO), he will intentionally employ the opposite approach and becomes notably more authoritative. In these instances, he purposely sprinkles in fancy jargon, leans back in his chair, uses a faster, sharper, pace in his speech, and maintains eye contact for greater lengths of time (see below for more advantages of being authoritative).

Greg Lamberty emphasizes the need for a soft approach, particularly with somatoform patients who have felt dismissed in previous medical encounters: "I walk carefully with words, because I realize the patient's emotional style might make an innocuous phrase from the neuropsychologist feel hurtful." To demonstrate this style, he shared the story of a veteran who came to see him after developing a tremor the day after a car accident. In the past, the patient had taken great offense to neuropsychologists and other specialists because he felt as though no one believed him.

> *I started by saying to the patient, "So you felt like the tremor began the day after the accident." Patient: "I didn't FEEL anything. It began the next day!" This patient also stated quite pointedly, "I don't know you, Doc, but docs have been very rude to me." I understood that if I said something this patient regarded as challenging, he would leave. Some people would be fine with saying, "I don't need to see this person. If he wants to go … Fine." But, I don't want to let him go. My choice is to see these cases as challenges: a challenge to not convey a "lack of respect," and a challenge to get information that might be useful or valid. The approach might be a little soft. I would readily acknowledge that. It's like getting a symptom validity test that's invalid. You could say, "This person is malingering," or you could say, "I wonder what that's about?"*

Of course, the words we use to communicate with patients should also match the patient's cognitive abilities.

> *I can't say, "Hey, dyslexic patient, read this book on coping with learning disabilities!" Or if someone has poor short-term memory, I don't want to use long paragraphs when I speak.*
>
> —*Christopher J. Nicholls, Ph.D.*

Slowing down one's rate of speech, and pausing frequently to check in and gauge the patient's understanding is another common communication technique amongst neuropsychologists that helps patients compensate for compromised attention, receptive language problems, and slowed processing speed. Many neuropsychologists comment directly on this aspect of their language to coach family members to do the same. For example, they might say something like, "Mr. Henderson, do.. you.. notice.. how.. slowly.. I ..am.. talking? Your.. wife.. will.. understand.. you.. better.. when.. you.. speak.. like.. this."

Modeling non-reactive repetition of information for families with a demented family member is also an important aspect of the communication subtext of the feedback session. Here is a common scenario: Following an emotionally draining half-hour conversation about driving in which the patient has been told he would have to turn in his keys, the patient says, "Okay, but my basic question is, I think I'm fine to drive. Do you have a problem with me driving?" This moment becomes an opportunity for the neuropsychologist to model a non-reactive way to address endlessly repeated questions. "Mr. Smith, yes, based on the testing you completed, it's not safe for you to drive. Here is a sheet of paper where I have written this information for you. You and your family can refer back to it when you have questions."

Authority

From the Freudian "Um-hmm," to the Rogerian "I hear you are frustrated that I am not sharing my thoughts," and the "one down approach" popular in family therapy, many psychological intervention techniques have pointedly avoided using a voice of authority with patients. The neuropsychological feedback session is a unique area in psychology where practitioners are often prescriptive. Depending on the circumstances, assuming an authoritative stance can facilitate a patient's ability to hear the feedback and act on recommendations. In fact, sometimes it is essential that we make an intentional effort to be more commanding.

> As psychologists we often tend to be fuzzy thinkers. We are often not authoritative enough, and might say something like, "Well, it's possible this might affect your driving…" Sometimes during neuropsychological feedback, patients need us to be authoritative. "You need to get a driving test, and I am going to make an appointment in three months to check in with you."
>
> —Gordon Chelune, Ph.D.

> You have to be authoritative. People view you as an authoritative figure, and you need to step up and be that. How authoritative I am depends on whose medical turf it is. I am comfortable being authoritative in my area of expertise. In other specialists' turf, for example, the integration of neuroradiological data, I will not assume an authoritative position.
>
> —Aaron Nelson, Ph.D.

Being authoritative allows the patient to trust in your opinions, to believe that they are working with an expert who knows what will be helpful to them or what constitutes a safe course of action.

> I make sure that if I feel like I need to take a stand, I take a stand. I am giving you my professional opinion based on data. And I tell you where I came up with my professional opinion. I present it in such a way that I am very confident about it. Being confident allows patients to feel okay about trusting in what I am telling them to do—because that's not always an easy thing for patients and parents to do. I will also tell them if I am less sure of a diagnosis, disposition, conclusion, etc., and why I am less sure.
>
> —E. Mark Mahone, Ph.D.

Finally, speaking confidently and with an authoritative presence is especially important when you are sharing emotionally loaded, or "bad" results.

> When you give difficult feedback, you need to be confident and as categorical as you can be. If you don't trust your findings and what you are saying, then patients and family members won't trust you.
>
> —Christopher Randolph, Ph.D.

ESTABLISHING TRUST WITHIN THE COMMUNITY

Establishing oneself as a trusted person in the community is another important way to increase your level of credibility. Robert Denney works in a prison hospital with an inmate population. He notes that many of the inmates assume people in a position of authority have ulterior motives when interacting with them.

> *I frequently have people tell me, "You aren't going to give me a transplant, because you want to get more money from keeping me on dialysis." Professionals in this setting can get a reputation for treating people with respect. It is also important to say something concrete about oneself, to further that trust. For example, I will tell patients, "I am a salaried employee. I have no vested interest. I will tell you this, I am going to be straight with you."*

Even in more traditional outpatient or inpatient settings, it is valuable to establish a positive community reputation.

> *I spend a considerable amount of time joining community organizations and giving talks. When other professionals refer patients to me, they can say with confidence that I understand the issues.*
>
> —*Monica Rivera-Mindt, Ph.D.*

This vote of confidence from the referral source can be an instrumental way to set the stage for trust between a clinician and the patient. It is this trust that allows the patient to see the neuropsychologist as an authority figure, and at times this first impression is even more important than the authority that you may convey through your interactions with the patient. Recognizing this point, Mark Barisa asks physicians to:

> *"Manage us up," when referring to our neuropsychology group. "Manage us up" is a business concept. When I refer to a pain person, I really play them up. I talk about how great that person is. It increases the likelihood they will show up. The strong endorsement of the person I am referring to tells them I value them, and I know who I am sending them to. It works the other way as well. We give workshops to referral sources, and say, "If you will set the stage for us, we will put on a show."*

SELF-DISCLOSURE

Are you going to be a blank screen upon which your patients project? Or are you going to sprinkle your feedback with personal anecdotes? Some clinicians are more comfortable with self-disclosure than others, but those who do use it point out that it can help them connect with a patient or family in ways that may not otherwise be available. For example, Mark Mahone shares with some families that he has a child with ADHD.

> *This allows me to talk about ADHD in a different way than if I didn't have a child with ADHD. I don't share too much information, but I do share with them that I understand the nature of a condition that can be with you throughout your life. Self-disclosure is a way of establishing credibility, and myself as a trusted member of the patient's "disorder community."*

In describing somatoform symptoms with patients, many clinicians use migraines as a way to demonstrate how they also experience psychological symptoms physically. "You know, I get migraines, and the first thing that I think when one hits me is, 'Oh! I must be stressed out!' I tend to be the type of person who feels my emotions through my body. The headache is a red flag to think, 'Okay, I need to work on my stress level.'" Self -disclosure in this instance can signal to patients that the discussion of somatic symptoms does not mean the clinician thinks they are "crazy." After all, their clinician has similar symptoms. Taking this disclosure one step further, Greg Lamberty tells some of his patients about when he developed intense shoulder pain at a board meeting just before his fortieth birthday:

> I was working with a group of neurologists at the time and was sure I was devel-oping multiple sclerosis. Of course, the symptoms passed with my birthday, and I realized in retrospect that I had been experiencing my own somatoform moment.

By sharing this personal experience, the patient is able to better appreciate and even normal-ize the fact that it is possible to experience emotions through physical symptoms in our body. It also allows them to be more receptive to the other conclusions and recommendations the clinician has to offer.

THE IMPACT OF APPEARANCE

Whether we like it or not, the age, or *perceived* age, of a clinician can significantly impact a patient's ability to trust them and therefore to accept their feedback. This can be especially important when clinicians are providing information that a patient does not want, or is not quite ready, to hear.

> How do you convince somatoform patients that you know what's going on? It helps to have gray hair. You need to have gravitas and it helps to be older. You are the expert. As an older neuropsychologist, I have no difficulty being taken seriously. It was harder when I was younger. As a younger practitioner, I would say to patients, "I'm young but I've been doing this for 10 years..." Now I don't need to say that. It's less work, because I'm taken seriously from the get-go.
> —Christopher Randolph, Ph.D.

Younger clinicians do not have the advantage of gray hair, and depending on their location and/or patient population, they may often receive comments about how young they are. How clinicians respond to a patient's concern about their apparent age, and therefore their presumed competence, is a critical opportunity to either establish trust or risk losing it. The following vignette offers a perfect example of this situation:

> An elderly woman walks into the consultation room, looks at the young neurop-sychologist, and utters the dreaded words, "You're so young!" This triggers a hum within the thought bubble of the neuropsychologist: "Yes! She's right! I am young. What am I doing here!? Wait, I have my Ph.D.! I'm fellowship trained! I have publications.... I've been practicing six years...." Some trainees and early clini-cians might find themselves responding, "Let me assure you, Mrs. Peters, that I am a fellowship trained neuropsychologist practicing for six years at the hospi-tal...." However, this kind of response can actually reduce the rapport with the

patient, who now offers an apology, but is still squinting at the neuropsychologist with some sense of distrust and now, embarrassment. A more experienced clinician might take an entirely different approach, "Oh my goodness! You just made my day! Why don't we go on in?" With these few deft words the challenge has been turned into an assumed compliment, and now the patient smiles and follows the clinician into the room.

While age cannot be altered, clothing can, and what one wears can also help establish trust. Think about the ubiquitous UNICEF tie printed with fanciful crayon drawings by children and worn by male child practitioners in almost every healthcare field. It communicates to parents, "I'm a serious professional, but your kid's going to like me." In the same manner, wearing a jacket and tie or a suit conveys authority to an adult patient before the clinician even introduces themselves. Cheryl Weinstein counsels her trainees to:

Look older, dress more formally. Sometimes I'll even suggest that they go buy a pair of glasses, even if they just have glass in them, and put them on.

In some situations, what a clinician wears is not only important to convey competency and authority, it can also be a critical way to establish oneself as a valid member of the patient's community. For example:

Non-military neuropsychologists who work in military medical centers are apt to don a white coat. "It's a culture of uniforms." This can also be a very masculine environment, so I and my female colleagues tend to avoid wearing skirts and dresses, choosing to wear pants instead under the lab coat.

—Laurie Ryan, Ph.D.

Social psychologists tell us that lasting impressions are clocked within seconds of meeting someone. Why not make those seconds work strategically to our clinical advantage?

CULTURAL CONSIDERATIONS

Throughout the book, we have incorporated pearls and strategies that are culturally specific within medical etiologies and patient populations. In this section we wanted to highlight some additional considerations for working with particular ethnic and socioeconomic groups. Our content is not exhaustive, and there are many topics that are not covered, but some clinicians shared perspectives in this area that warranted their own heading.

The decision to assess individuals from less familiar cultural or socioeconomic backgrounds can be complex, and occurs well before the feedback session begins. Neuropsychologists in urban centers might have the option of referring to a colleague who has a high degree of competence in the particular culture. There are times, though, when no culturally competent colleague is available due to the nature of the referral or a rural setting. Even in these instances, some neuropsychologists are reluctant to evaluate patients unless they are totally culturally competent and have good norms. Unfortunately, this raises the risk that a patient or patient population will be unable to access necessary medical treatment. Many other clinicians take a different stance on the issue:

My feeling is that if a patient needs an evaluation, and there is no one else to do it, I am willing to assess the patient, recognizing the limitations of the norms and cultural factors.

—Paul Craig, Ph.D.

Under these circumstances, acknowledging one's limitations can also be a useful way to facilitate trust and further support the feedback process.

We don't need to walk into feedback sessions with complete a priori awareness of the cultural implications of our message. That would be impossible. Neuropsychologists are best able to pitch their message when they are open to engaging in a dialogue and asking questions about their patients' culture. It's important for someone from a different background to be okay with not knowing everything. So even if I suspect I know a different culture well, it's important to give the patient a chance to tell me. I will invite them to do so by directly asking, "How's this in your culture?" Or, "From your background, how do you deal with this?" When I am on their turf, I find out about their turf.

—Tony Wong, Ph.D.

Cultural sensitivity for the use of language

When working with Latinos, Monica Rivera-Mindt begins assessments by asking what their preferred language is. Because members of the family may attend the feedback session without having come to previous appointments, the question of preferred language should be raised again, even if it was discussed during the interview. Even when feedback sessions are presented in English, an understanding of, and a respect for, the family's primary language can facilitate the process in many ways.

I might give feedback primarily in English, but there are certain phrases/things that are easier to explain in Spanish. It's hard to say why, but it is easier to explain emotional experience in Spanish. Idioms of distress might be easier to discuss in Spanish. And it might feel less threatening to use such idioms, for example "ataques de nervios," which is culturally specific and often associated with depression.

The use of culturally sensitive language and the awareness of cultural norms is equally important with Alaskan Natives.

In the Midwest culture in which I grew up, people speak until they are comfortable, then they can be quiet together. In general, Alaska Natives are quiet until such time that they are comfortable. Then they speak. The pace of conversation is different. When I stop talking, I need to leave more time for them to answer, rather than jumping in and rephrasing the question with the assumption they don't understand it or need it restated. There is a longer pause between people communicating—bouncing the ball back and forth—than most people from my cultural heritage are comfortable with.

—Paul Craig, Ph.D.

Even decisions regarding when and how to use titles can vary depending upon the culture. For example, Monica Rivera-Mindt emphasizes that, in Latino culture, "La Doctora" is a very formal role; use of language with this group is formal and very polite. There is an expectation for an authoritative, prescriptive delivery style. In this context, use of the formal title is expected, and helpful to the process.

When using translators

Although most neuropsychologists will try to refer to a clinician who speaks the patient's language, in some cases this is not possible. In those situations, it is helpful to clarify prior to the feedback session who will be translating. Monica Rivera-Mindt notes that for first-generation immigrants, children are often taken to medical visits to translate. Thus she might find a child walking into the feedback session, ready to help his parents understand the findings. However, a professional translator, or another adult family member is preferable, as the content of the feedback session may be inappropriate for children.

> *Sometimes kids who are more acculturated will be expected to come to feedback sessions to translate. It's delicate to disrupt that processes. I am able to speak Spanish directly with my Latino patients, so I can redirect the child from the room. I usually say something like, "Oh! I should have told you, this is the part where I have to speak alone with your mother. This is the way we do it."*

Even with the assistance of a translator, it can be difficult to convey the full meaning of our findings to families who are recent immigrants to the United States, or who are less acculturated. For this reason, Karen Wills finds the use of models and pictures particularly important when working with families who need an interpreter.

> *I see a lot of Hmong families and Somali families. I don't speak their language, and have no idea what the interpreter is saying. I try to do a lot of the feedback with visual aids. I make pictures, and then ask the families through the interpreter, "Did you get that? Can you give me an example of when you see that?"*

Similarly, even when neuropsychologists and patients speak the same language, cultural or socioeconomic factors may create a language barrier. Jim Irby stresses the need to communicate to patients and families in a language that is familiar to them:

> *I try to use their language, and listen carefully to what's important to them. And I address that in feedback. The key is to use their language, not our language. When I do need to use more technical language, I will reference, "Now the fancy word for this is...."*

Unique cultural issues associated with rapport

Many clinicians who work with Latino patients commented on the predominance of traditional family roles. Care should be taken to convey respect, especially to the male family figurehead. At the same time, those traditional family hierarchies may be stressed by parents' having to rely on their more acculturated children. Understanding the dynamics that may be in play with each patient facilitates a clinician's ability to establish trust and maintain rapport over time. Another consideration in working with Latino patients is *"familismo,"* or the importance of family connections, which can extend to community members' *"personalismo."* Monica Rivera-Mindt explains:

> *The beginning of a neuropsychological assessment with a patient or family may be very formal. By end of the feedback session the boundaries often shift. At this point the patient sees you as someone who is trying to help him or her. You are now seen as an ally. If they see you in the community, they might also be very warm. They will still address you as La Doctora, but they can be VERY warm. People might want to hug you or embrace, bring food. When the boundaries shift, you have to go with that and respect that things are now a little different.*

When working with immigrant families, Monica Rivera-Mindt also emphasized,

> *I don't ask questions about immigration status. For example, I would never ask, "Are you legal?" unless it is an immigration case. But, I will ask, "Where were you born?"*

Cultural issues associated with low socioeconomic status

Neuropsychologists practicing in high socioeconomic communities have the luxury of making recommendations for services and treatments that might not be available or accessible in less affluent communities. For example, feedback for a child struggling with dyslexia in a wealthy suburb might include recommendations for tutors trained in scientifically based reading programs. Such tutors may not be available in lower socioeconomic communities, or affordable for particular families. Jennifer Turek Queally reports that her own blue-collar background has left her with a strong practical approach to feedback with low-socioeconomic-status families. This awareness leads to different emphases, depending upon the needs of the family. For example, she makes an effort to be cognizant of a family's resources and spends more time in feedback addressing how they can access available resources.

In addition to the variability associated with socioeconomic status, resources can also be extremely limited in rural communities. An occupational therapist might not exist to give a dementia patient a driving evaluation. There also may be no local child psychologist who can provide cognitive behavioral therapy (CBT) to an anxious seven-year-old, even if his parents could afford co-pays.

> *Since I practice in Alaska, I see people in bush villages that might have only two teachers, no speech language pathologists, and no nurses, not to mention a physician. In these cases, I believe that we have to couch the recommendations in the context of realistic resources that can be used to implement those recommendations. In Boston, a neuropsychologist might think about the issue of driving. In the Alaska bush, the safety issue might be using a chainsaw or four-wheeler. We have to say to ourselves, are our recommendations relevant to this individual's activities of daily living?*
>
> —*Paul Craig, Ph.D.*

APPROACHING EMOTIONS

Raising the topic of mood disorders, or discussing the interplay of patients' symptoms and stressors in the context of feedback, is a delicate process in nearly all instances. Clinicians guide the conversation through a potential minefield, careful not to offend while attempting to be clear and direct. Navigating these conversations when one is less familiar with the patient's cultural or socioeconomic context can be even more difficult. Tony Wong provided this advice:

> *I actually come from the inner city, but it's been a long time. Whether I like it or not, I am now middle class. And not only middle class, but a psychologist and neuropsychologist. All this stuff about emotion is old hat and non-threatening to talk about. With lower socioeconomic patients two things go on that I try to pay attention to:*
>
> *First, there's a built in adaptive paranoia of professionals. They are suspicious, wary, concerned about how people above them might look down upon them, use information against them, or use information in a patronizing, dismissive way. So when I have a Low SES situation, I approach the issues more carefully and slowly. And I take a long time to explain things.*
>
> *Second, with emotional issues, I am sensitive to the possibility that they may be afraid that they will perceived to be crazy. With some cultures, and lower SES, it's nice to couch it in a biological explanation. It's often more acceptable to have something wrong with your brain than your mind. With traditional Asian culture, psychological issues are generally taboo. Those things raise a lot of anxiety. You have to handle them very carefully.*
>
> *For patients from a European middle-class American, young background, I might be more quick to recommend counseling or psychotherapy. It doesn't seem as aversive to them. For someone who is older, from a lower SES background, or from another cultural background, particularly Asian or Hispanic/ Latino, I would also broach it more carefully; I'll float it by them to see if they might be open to [it]. If they are resistant, I will ask them, "Does that have to do with your cultural background, is that where some of your reluctance come from?"*
>
> *I won't back down in terms of what I think patients need, but I will be flexible in terms of how the need can be met. I might say something like, "You know, this is a problem we need to address. I am willing to work with you in terms of how to best address this. But it wouldn't be right to just let it go."*
>
> —*Tony Wong, Ph.D.*

EXPERIENCE OF DEPENDENCE AND INDEPENDENCE

Symptoms of mild dementia might not generate much stress in one family, while another extended family is sent into crisis when Mom is unable to handle her own finances. Part of the differences relating to this tolerance stems from the presence or absence of built-in systems to pick up the slack when one family member becomes less functional. Do the grown children all live within a three-mile radius, in a well-connected community? Or are the children scattered across several states, with no one within two hours' drive able to assist? Whether or not family members are physically in close proximity, a patient's cultural background may also dictate family members' perceptions of their roles vis-à-vis their increasing dependence. Awareness of these cultural expectations can assist families in developing a care plan.

Molly Warner's experience has been that cultural differences in role expectations regarding a family member with disabilities can be significant. For example:

> *In general, Hispanic families will care for disabled children, sometimes without a goal of independence where more could be achieved; in contrast, many European American cultures will have a goal of independence, even when that isn't necessarily appropriate. Understanding cultural expectations, by asking questions about how dependence versus independence is handled in the patient's culture, can facilitate care planning.*

Understanding our patients' cultural backgrounds and associated approach to medical-related issues, psychological functioning, and dependency is an essential component of any effective neuropsychological practice. These pearls are a strong reminder of this facet of our practice. More importantly, they encourage us to ask questions whenever we are working with someone outside of our own culture, so as to strengthen our connections with the family as well as our neuropsychological conceptualizations and recommendations.

REFERENCE

Russell RL. Social communication impairments: pragmatics. *Pediatr Clin North Am.* Jun 2007;54(3):483–506, vi.

II Putting Feedback to Work

5 Putting Feedback to Work with Patients from Multiple Populations

(countinued)

MANY FEEDBACK METAPHORS and strategies can be used broadly, across multiple patient populations. Regardless of the specific disease process or presenting concern, these pearls can be utilized to connect with patients and families, introduce/demystify assessment results, bridge cultures and religions, explain general cognitive constructs such as memory and attention, and introduce recommendations.

DEVELOPING RELATIONSHIPS WITH PATIENTS AND FAMILIES

Many neuropsychologists comment that even our own extended family members do not know exactly what we do for a living. More often than not our work is also a mysterious process to members of the public. Therefore, an important task is helping patients and their families understand how we can be helpful to them and how they might rely on us in the future. It is also important to put patients and their families at ease about their decision to come in, diffuse common barriers to "hearing" feedback, and to create bonds that ensure clinicians are viewed as trusted, long-term members of the care team. The following are particularly adroit methods of accomplishing these tasks.

CONNECTING WITH THE PATIENT/FAMILY

Affirming parents' instincts

- o *"You've come to the right place. This is exactly the type of thing that we do well, and these are the questions that we know how to answer. And today, I think we have a really clear answer for you." (I want them to leave the session feeling informed, to hear my confidence in the "understandableness" of the child's problem, and to feel like they came to the right place.)*

  —*Steve Hughes, Ph.D.*

- o *"You had the right instincts. You know your child well. When you came in, you were concerned about Sam. The testing shows us you were right to be concerned."*

  —*Robin Hilsabeck, Ph.D.*

Establishing a long-term relationship

- o *"Our relationship doesn't stop once you have the report. See me as a dentist. You will want to come in once a year for a reading checkup. I want to be available for you, and I am happy to stay on and be involved as much as you want me to. I am here to be a resource for you as you adjust to this information" (or have to deal with school issues, etc.).*

  —*Steven Guy, Ph.D.*

- o *"I'm going to start providing you with information now. Some of it may feel right, some may not. You can come back in a month and tell me what you think. Be critical—I may not be right."*

  —*Cheryl Weinstein, Ph.D.*

Normalizing the presenting symptom(s)

- *"The good news here is that these are relatively common problems and we know what to do. I want you to know that while your child is extraordinary in his own right, what we are seeing here is exceptionally garden-variety stuff"* (e.g., this is a garden-variety of ADHD, reading disability, etc). *"It's been mysterious, but this problem is understood, and we can point you in the right direction for good treatment."*
  —*Steve Hughes, Ph.D.*

Contextualizing a history of conflicting diagnoses

Parents may feel frustrated that their child has been given several different diagnoses over time. This helps them to understand why their child's diagnosis has changed, and avoids a situation in which the family leaves the assessment thinking, "OK, one more assessment, one more diagnosis, which is the REAL one?"

- *"Look, when your child was young, they said that he was slow at motor development. Why did they say that? Because that's what kids do at that age. They develop motor skills—crawling and walking. Then they said that he had a communication problem. Why? Because that's what kids do at that age—they develop language. Then there was an 'attention problem.' Then a 'learning disorder.' What they were doing was 'pieces parts' approach. They were diagnosing a problem with what ever the developmental task was at the time. 'Pieces parts' isn't going to help him. We need to roll this up. Let's talk about the whole child."*
  —*Tom Boll, Ph.D.*

Encouraging questions from patients and families

When patients don't know much, they stop asking questions, when they should be asking *more* questions. Malcolm Gladwell pointed out that low SES people, who are insecure about their knowledge, will ask minimal questions. People with more knowledge, will get to ask more questions. If people aren't asking questions, I will give them lots of information.

- *"Let me give you some background information here."*
  —*Jim Scott, Ph.D.*

CREATING A THERAPEUTIC ATMOSPHERE

When working with children who have serious medical conditions, parents frequently know at some level that their child will not experience a "good" outcome. They may not realize that the neuropsychological assessment is a place where they can express their grief at receiving difficult news, or their distress as the implications of a longstanding diagnosis becomes clear when new developmental phases are reached. Creating a therapeutic environment helps patients feel comfortable enough to share their concerns or to be receptive to our findings.

Giving parents a space to grieve

Following severe TBI, or any other life threatening injury or illness that affects cognition, the fact that the child is still alive can make parents hesitant to grieve for their lost child, including the future they envisioned for that particular child. It's important to give parents permission to grieve. This is really a subtext of the feedback session: to help the parents acknowledge that they have lost the child they thought they had. Grieving is an important step in acknowledging where the child is now and moving the family forward. On an inpatient unit, this is something that can occur over multiple sessions.

> o *"Your child was not the only one who was injured. You were also injured, just not physically. There needs to be a healing process for you as well."*
> —*Michael Kirkwood, Ph.D.*

This pearl arises out of a postdoctoral fellowship at the Yale child study center, where I was supervised by psychoanalysts. What parents need from the professional neuropsychologist is a segue—a way to step into the nature of their loss.

> o *"Well, she has so many strengths. And here's what they are … but you know, as I looked at the school records you provided, and as I looked at her performance on academic achievement tests, it looks like something's changed in math. Has there been a change in math?" (Mom—"Yeah, she can't do it, it doesn't work").*
>
> *"That's exactly what the results show. It doesn't work the way it used to." (As soon as you use that phrase, "it doesn't work the way it used to," you have opened up the discussion about loss and grief. The child, who was perfect, is now somehow damaged). "Well, it just seems like you probably have some feelings about that" (and that's all it takes to open up).*
>
> *(The next step in the conversation.…) "It is a change, and that's sad …" (pause). "Here's what we can do. What we need to talk about is how we are going to adapt to the change, and what steps you can take to bring about some type of improvement with the conditions as they are now."*
> —*Paul Kaufman, Ph.D.*

Scaffolding language to help patients express concerns

Patients and family members might not have the language to express their concerns. Clinicians can supply language without "putting words in patient's mouths" by introducing hypothetical concerns based on what other, similar patients have shared.

> o *"Some teenagers" (people prior to transplant surgery, mothers of autistic children, etc.) "are concerned about.…"*
> —*Marc Norman, Ph.D.*

Complimenting patients on their resiliency

> ***Something to consider:*** *one of my postdoctoral fellowship mentors, Paul Satz, used to simply tell patients at the opportune moment, "You're a survivor, then, aren't you?" The reaction, therapeutic engagement, and "patient satisfaction" of this moment was something to behold*
>
> —*Jeff Cory, Ph.D.*

Addressing patient distress during the feedback session

> *People can become very anxious at feedback sessions. When this becomes apparent, I try not to leave until I have identified why they look anxious. "You look concerned now. Let's talk about that … what do you feel is the best-case scenario and worst-case scenario?"*
>
> —*Marc Norman, Ph.D.*

For many children with disabilities, or adults who struggle cognitively, praise is something they seldom hear. Hearing praise that is concretely anchored to what we have discovered about their effort, personality, and abilities can be particularly powerful and therapeutic when coming from a doctor that has ushered them through a multi-hour assessment process.

Praising the child

Clinicians can take praise one step further by making a personality attribution. Even if the attribution is not how the child or family sees the child, clinicians are offering a positive alternate narrative, or reinforcing an existing narrative. This is also great to model for parents. The template is: compliment … you're the type of person who.…

> o *"Wow, great job finishing all those tests. You're the type of kid who keeps trying, even when things are hard."*
>
> —*Karen Postal, Ph.D.*

SETTING THE STAGE FOR FEEDBACK

As discussed in Chapter 3, prior to presenting results, many clinicians take time to set the stage about how the feedback session will be structured, before informing patients and family members about what the tests measured and how diagnoses were reached. The following are examples of how to effectively communicate the context of assessment results, without losing patients to jargon or excessive length.

Reassuring with good news

It is often helpful to let patients know right away when the news is good. Otherwise, their anxiety can get in the way of their ability to hear whatever information is given in the beginning of the session.

> o *"I want to go through some of the results of the evaluation. I'm sure you will have some questions. Let me say right away that I think things turned out very well. We can go over details, but overall, the news is good."*
>
> —*Greg Lamberty, Ph.D.*

A lot of kids come in fearing that they are stupid. It is important to find a simple way, up front, to tell them that they are not.

> o *"Just to let you know, the bottom line is, you're not stupid."*
>
> —*Keith Owen Yeates, Ph.D.*

Responding to the patient's presenting concern(s)

During the initial interview, it's helpful to ask patients and family members what they think is the cause of the problem. This lets you know where the patient and family are around the potential diagnoses. For example, it's good to not have to be the first person to mention Alzheimer disease. The family's conjectures can then be revisited during the feedback session.

> o *"Do you know when you said you thought that this was Alzheimer disease at our first meeting? I'm pleased to be able to tell you this doesn't look like Alzheimer's."*
>
> —*Richard Naugle, Ph.D.*

Validating patient concerns about memory

> o *"Do you remember when you first came in here? You told me you were having some trouble with your memory. Well, you were right. It's really good that you were proactive and came here … Let's talk about your memory.…"*
>
> —*Robin Hilsabeck, Ph.D.*

Acknowledging how tiring testing can be

> o *"We wore you out with the testing. We were worn out too. Let's go over the results."*
>
> —*David E. Tupper, Ph.D.*

Engaging children in a dialogue about their abilities

In the beginning of a feedback session, I start with a description of the child's strengths. Then I pivot to weakness. To do this, I enlist the child in identifying their own weakness. This is really a dialogue. In order to do this well, you have to remember what it is like to be a child.

> o *"Do you remember when we did the thing with the blocks? Well, I think we really found that was an area of strength. You really enjoyed that, and you really did well. I know too that there were some places that were harder. Can you tell me one*

of the tests that was harder? Or, one of the tests that you didn't like? I think you're right. I think that's a challenge, and we might be able to help you."

—*Paul Kaufmann, JD, Ph.D.*

Inviting parents to help shape the feedback message

The answer to this question is informative. Parents are not just being asked for what they want me to say, they are being asked to reiterate what they have heard. It's a very good way to ensure the parents themselves have gotten the message.

o *"I am going to speak with your child now about these results. Is there anything that you want me to be sure to tell them?"*

—*Steve Hughes, Ph.D.*

"Wondering out loud" to engage patients

I do therapy as well, and use many stock therapeutic phrases. In a neuropsychological feedback session, I often say the same thing that I might in a psychotherapy session, which is usually "wondering out loud" with the patient. Of course in a neuropsychological feedback session, I have more data.

o *"You think maybe? You think maybe this might be a problem for you? The test data suggests that to me."*

—*Jim Irby, Ph.D.*

This is an indirect way of asking the patients for feedback on the evaluation process. Asking directly to make sure that nothing is being missed. You never know what they will say. Every once in a while patients and family will say something, or ask a question that will take things in a different direction.

o *"Does this sound right? Does this seem to be what you're seeing?"*

—*David E. Tupper, Ph.D.*

EXPLAINING THE TESTING PROCESS AND GOALS

The rationale for comprehensive testing

o *"When your mother was tested" (or "when you were tested") "what we did was take a tour of your brain. Now we know what's working and what's not working as well...."*

—*Susan McPherson, Ph.D.*

o *"Everyone has a cognitive landscape that has peaks and valleys. The reason we do a full battery is that it gives us a lot of detail about the peaks and valleys of your child's cognitive landscape. Now that we've done that, we are going to take a while and describe that cognitive landscape."*

—*Steve Hughes, Ph.D.*

Why does testing take so long?

Sometimes patients, family members (and even insurance companies) will ask, why does testing take so long?

o *"Well, we're measuring the most complicated thing in the universe. What's more complicated than your child's brain? We can't assess that with a short cut."*
—Michael Joschko, Ph.D.

Giving parents a chance to take the tests

During the feedback session, I like to have the child give one of the tests to the parents. This helps to stimulate a conversation about the tests and what they measure.

o *"Johnny is going to give you a language test, so we can all be on the same page about what skills we are talking about. Ok, Johnny...."*
—Michael Joschko, Ph.D.

EXPLAINING THE NORMAL CURVE

Height metaphor for the normal curve

This is a very helpful analogy for explaining the normal curve, without an emphasis on "higher is better," or saying that lower necessarily represents a disease process or deficit.

o *"How tall is the average American woman? 5'6. But most women are between 5'3 and 5'10. There aren't a lot of women who are much smaller or much taller. They would be down there, or up here. Ok, so here's this curve. Most women are in here, the average range. But some are really short, there down here. Just because it falls out of the average range, doesn't mean it's a disease. Let's take finger tapping. Just because you're really fast, does it mean you're better? Not really. You might be better at touch-typing, but...."*
—Christopher J. Nicholls, Ph.D.

ACKNOWLEDGING THE LIMITATIONS OF TESTING

Addressing the limitations of the neuropsychological testing process in the beginning of the session can increase a patient's' capacity to hear feedback about their abilities—and their difficulties. Taking the time to address this issue before patients bring it up on their own can "inoculate" against the whole testing process being dismissed, particularly when patients lack awareness. In some situations, neuropsychological testing may not be able to clearly measure deficits, particularly with subtle executive dysfunction. In that case, addressing the limitations of the tests serves as a needed caveat in addressing the ultimate diagnosis.

o *"These tests, now they're not perfect. That's why I spend time getting to know you. I don't just go by the test scores. Some people may have always had problems with math. Or they just aren't good test takers. The tests aren't perfect and so I don't want to misinterpret them. But they give us an idea of your both your weaknesses and your strengths. I want you to have this information, so you can make good decisions for yourself."*

—*Jim Irby, Ph.D.*

o *"We are testing in an unnatural environment. We're not testing in a grocery store, or classroom, or worksite, so we might not be able to pick up on the problem."*

—*Erin D. Bigler, Ph.D.*

We do a lousy job measuring executive functions. We give patients instructions, organize, and prompt them. Because of this, a patient's challenges with executive functions or memory problems may not be well measured in our assessments. The following helps to address this issue and can also be a great segue to help patients understand the rationale for compensatory strategies.

o *"All I can tell you is that at least within the context of a structure and standard-ized testing situation, your memory appears to be okay. That doesn't mean you may not experience occasional lapses in your memory in day-to-day life due to stressors or having lots going on. What I can tell you is that it's not necessarily an ongoing 'always' problem. And that's a good sign.*

What we need to do is explore a little more, what are the circumstances where it is hard for you, and maybe there are things you can do to structure your life in a way where you are experiencing less of that kind of interference—simple things you can do to relieve the burden on your memory."

—*Gordon Chelune, Ph.D.*

OFFERING HOPE AND NORMALIZING FINDINGS

Many patients respond catastrophically to their diagnosis. Parents may also respond to their child's diagnosis with a feeling of hopelessness. This simple statement can frame the discussion of recommendations.

o *"You need to know that this is not a deal breaker. Here's what people who have this problem can do."*

—*Steve Hughes, Ph.D.*

o *Some individuals feel limited and demeaned by the diagnostic process. In many instances I say, "Your diagnosis is not a red light. You should see it as a way of understanding things—and then manage them. The last thing I want you to do is become a patient. I want you to understand that you have a problem and then I want you to figure out ways that you're going to manage that problem. I want you to also understand that you are a person much more than a patient. You have a responsibility to yourself to put this problem in its place."*

—*Margaret O'Connor, Ph.D.*

EXPLAINING MEMORY

Memory deficits are common across many neuropsychological syndromes. The following are helpful feedback techniques that work well for a broad cross-section of patients.

Library metaphor for memory

This metaphor is useful for differentiating memory problems due to storage vs. retrieval:

o *"Different people have memory problems for different reasons. It's like going into a library. Sometimes the book has been checked out—it isn't there. Sometimes the book is just mis-shelved and it takes a while to find it. If you get cues, then it helps to figure out where that book is shelved."*

—*Gordon Chelune, Ph.D.*

You can also expand the library metaphor to differentiate encoding vs. retrieval deficits.

o *"Imagine that your brain is like a library, and making a new memory is like putting a new book in that library. When you need to remember something ('pull it out'), it's a little like asking the librarian of your brain to go back through the stacks of books, find the book and come back to the front of the library with it.*

Forgetfulness or 'memory loss' is like an 'empty-handed librarian.' If the librarian can't find the book, it may be that (a) the book is nowhere in the library at all, or (b) that it is in the library somewhere and may have been filed on the wrong shelf, or even tossed in a closet or on the floor, making it hard to find. In the latter case, the 'book' is actually in there, but it just can't be 'pulled out.'

If cues and reminders serve to 'jog' your memory—sort of like giving the librarian a choice between three books, one of which is the one that was being searched for—or if such reminders make the 'light bulb (of memory) go off,' like 'oh, that's right!' we can be confident that a memory was formed (i.e., the book got into the library), but it just wasn't easy for the brain's 'librarian' to pull it out."

When memories are not being successfully made, we call that amnesia, and it means 'there's no book on the shelf.' When a person experiences amnesia (that is, the book never gets into the library successfully), it typically means that a part of the brain, in fact the part that is disrupted first in Alzheimer disease, is not functioning well. But when a person is experiencing retrieval impairment (i.e., the book/memory is 'in there, but I can't get it out' without cues or reminders), a different part of the brain is most likely dysfunctional, often involving the frontal lobes and their connections, deep down in the brain, to other parts of the brain." Understanding where the breakdown in memory formation and recall is occurring in the brain (i.e., why the librarian comes back empty-handed) can be very important in determining what areas are not working properly, and relatedly, what to do about it and what to expect in the patient's future.

—*Jeff Cory, PhD*

The impact of memory/attention deficits on marriage

Memory and/or attention problems in one spouse can create significant marital problems. All you have to do in feedback is lay this out, and they understand it. You've really cut out a lot of reasons to fight.

○ *"Have you two been having arguments about 'he said/she said?' Now, whenever you have one of these 'he said/she said's,' I have to tell you"* (to patient) *"you're wrong, and your spouse is right.*

"I'll explain what's happening. She's talking too fast. And you only hear part of it. Here's an example: This is Friday night. 'Honey, tomorrow is Saturday. I am going to meet Marybeth. We'll have lunch at Nordstrom's. I need to find a dress for her daughter's wedding. I will probably get home at 4:00, but there is a possibility I will get stuck and not be home until 6:00. Now the Smiths are coming for dinner. Can you put the potatoes in the oven at 5?'

Now it's Saturday at 5:30. You're pacing and in a rage. 'Where have you been?!' 'She said she would come at 4, but might be as late as 6....' You are outraged. Then she looks at the oven, which you haven't turned on, and she is outraged!! But you only heard the first part of what she said: 'I'll probably get home at 4:00.'"
                                                                    —*Muriel D. Lezak, Ph.D.*

Explaining the impact of attention on memory

This is a good pearl for the "worried well." It helps explain the attention factor involved when you forget why you went to the kitchen.

○ *"You know how you go into the kitchen to get something and by the time you go into the next room, you don't remember what you went for? So you get up out of your living room chair to go get a glass of milk and you step into the kitchen, which is the very next room. Meanwhile, some other thought has occurred to you. And then you get to the kitchen and you were not able to hold onto the thought that brought you out of your chair in the first place."*
                                                                    —*Roger Cohen, Ph.D.*

○ *"Look, you scored so well on your memory tests, but not on the attention tests. So it's not your memory."* (Turns to spouse, using a slow, slow voice) *"Talk ... with ... your ... husband ... at a slow pace ... this is what you need to do. And tell your teenage children, this is how you talk to your dad. If something is very important, you will need to repeat it."*
                                                                    —*Muriel D. Lezak, Ph.D.*

○ *"Memory can fail in everyday life, but may not reflect a real neurocognitive deficit or be reflected on formal testing. The flood of information we are all faced with every day may be distracting you. If you are distracted, you won't be paying attention; then it will feel like a memory problem."*
                                                                    —*Munro Cullum, Ph.D.*

PEARLS TO EXPLAIN SLOWED/INEFFICIENT PROCESSING

o *"Your problem is not stupidity. It's inefficiency. Your processing is slowed."*

—*Muriel D. Lezak, Ph.D.*

Computer metaphor for slowed processing

o *"This might help to explain the changes in your brain from the (CVA, TBI, etc.). Think about an enormous, totally superhumongous computer. It fills the whole room, it's so big. Imagine that someone comes in with a little metal hammer. They knock out a little connection here, and one over here, and a couple over here. And then they run the computer. And a few things have changed. One, because there are these disconnections, things are short-circuited. The message has a longer route. It has to bypass the short circuit. So the whole process has slowed down. Another change is that almost everything the computer produces will be absolutely accurate. Except when it is not. And you will never know whether the answer that comes out is the right answer."*

—*Muriel D. Lezak, Ph.D.*

Younger patients respond well to computer metaphors. This pearl helps explain slowness in processing and how it affects memory function.

o *"Your hard drive is fine. All the information you've always stored is still there. Some of your software—how you accessed that information—might have changed a little now since the injury/illness. It might take you a little longer to run from one point in the program to another—to retrieve the information—but the information is still there. You need to give the CPU longer to process."*

—*Munro Cullum, Ph.D.*

For cases with medical conditions that have diffuse effects on functioning (commonly, slowed processing or mild attention deficits with intermittent errors), I give the analogy of a computer that has a virus.

o *"Following the" (fill in the condition, such as TBI), "sometimes you will notice that there are some changes in how efficiently your brain is working. It's like a computer with a virus. Just like a computer with a virus—the machine is working, but sometimes it will take longer, and you may have glitches now and then (e.g., the screen will freeze, etc.). It's best to be sensitive to these needs, with realistic expectations, and give your brain time to 'reset' when needed, instead of just hitting the 'enter' key repeatedly out of frustration.*

"In other words, you will need to be sensitive to rising frustration, and take breaks when needed, rather than pushing ahead when things are going poorly. Of course, you can still use a computer with a virus, as long are you are sensitive to adapting when necessary, rather than just 'shutting down' out of frustration and failing to attempt certain activities."

—*Lisa Riemenschneider, Psy.D.*

Walking with a small child metaphor for slowed processing speed

o *"Have you ever walked with a small child? You are just taking a leisurely pace, but that little kid is almost at a run to keep up with you. That is similar to your husband's brain right now and it is why he likely has problems keeping up in conversations or in busy environments. While your brain can easily keep up a fairly rapid pace, his brain has to work much harder just to keep up. As such, he is likely going to trip over some details just as that small child sometimes trips over things as he or she is trying to keep up the same pace as you."*

—*Andrea Zartman, Ph.D.*

EXPLAINING EXECUTIVE FUNCTION AND FRONTAL IMPAIRMENT

Additional pearls for explaining executive function can be found in Chapter 7: ADHD.

Explaining "Can't vs. Won't" in the context of executive dysfunction

Often family members feel that cognitive symptoms are essentially about lack of motivation. This is true particularly with ADHD populations, or individuals who are a few years status post-traumatic brain injury. Addressing the distinction between "can't and won't" during a feedback session allows a productive conversation to begin. (For other pearls regarding "can't vs. won't," see Chapter 7: ADHD.)

o *"Everyone is frustrated by John's trouble at work and home. One of the purposes of the assessment was to try to sort out 'can't' versus 'won't;' to help sort out whether John can't do these things or whether he won't."*

—*Paul Craig, Ph.D.*

Symphony conductor metaphor for executive function

o *"The brain is organized like a symphony orchestra. The back of the brain has the sections of the orchestra. Just like you have horns and strings, in the brain you have visuoperception, language, and sense of touch. The front of the brain is the conductor. The conductor starts and stops the orchestra. If someone makes a mistake, it is the conductor who catches it and corrects it. This is where you have self-awareness. The conductor is responsible for starting and stopping. If the orchestra starts to play before the constructor says 'go,' we call that impulsiveness. If the band keeps playing after the conductor says 'stop'—we call that perseveration."*

—*Barbara J. Schrock, Ph.D.*

Cleaning an attic metaphor for executive dysfunction

o *"Say you inherit a house, and you walk into the attic—and it's so full of stuff. You feel demoralized, and are like, 'I don't even know where to begin.' It's like that for your husband when getting dressed in the morning—just on a different level. 'I don't even know where to begin. Do I start with a pant leg?'"*

—*Yana Suchy, Ph.D.*

Dog and a tennis ball metaphor for executive function

This is an effective way of explaining stimulus-bound frontal behavior.

o *"It's kind of like, your dog is going over to his bowl, and he has this goal, 'Okay, I'm going to go get a drink.' But then he sees the edge of a tennis ball and 'ching!' He grabs the ball. That happens with people too when the frontal lobe is damaged. They are doing a task, and then see something else, and 'Ching!' the new stimulus drives their behavior."*

—*Yana Suchy, Ph.D.*

When a patient with severe frontal impairment can't let go of an object, people have a hard time understanding what is going on, and sometimes even the therapists who are working with the patient may be confused. The expectation is—if you want to do it, of course you will. So the behavior of a patient with a frontal lobe injury is misinterpreted as being stubborn or oppositional.

o *"Think about when you play ball with your dog. The dog comes over, and he wants you to take the ball and throw it. But he's still holding the ball. It's as though he can't let go—ah-ah-ah-ah. You know he wants you to throw the ball, he enjoys going after the ball, but he just can't let go of it. Just like with that dog playing ball, there is a disconnect between what your son wants to do, and what his motor system ends up doing. He is holding the walker, and wants to let go of it, but can't seem to let go."*

—*Yana Suchy, Ph.D.*

Facilitating caregiver empathy for impaired reasoning

When you have someone who is not able to reason, because of TBI, CVA, etc., their judgment is impaired. So they just get more and more upset when you push the issue. You have to help the family recognize when they've stumbled into a situation where reasoning is not working, and then how to shift their focus to their emotional tone. For example, I recently had a woman who kept putting her amnestic and confabulating husband on the spot. She kept asking, almost sarcastically, "Do you really believe that?" In her way, she was trying to reason with him. Of course, he had no awareness he was confabulating, and they both just got more and more agitated. Once she understood the severity of his memory problems and how they both got upset when she kept trying to reason him out of his confabulations, it was really helpful.

o *"You can't reason someone out of a position they didn't reason themselves into in the first place. He doesn't realize what he's saying and he can't reason along with you. If you have tried to reason with him and its not working, take a few deep breaths and change the subject."*

—*Jim Irby, Ph.D.*

OFFERING RECOMMENDATIONS AND COMPENSATORY STRATEGIES

Cheryl Weinstein recalls Edith Kaplan saying that anybody can talk about deficits, "anybody. You don't even have to be a neuropsychologist for that. But what are the conditions under which you can recoup? Where are the strengths—what mechanisms are we seeing as neuropsychologists that the patients are already using as compensatory strategies? And what can we suggest?" Offering compensatory strategies that are tailored to patient's strengths is empowering:

> o *People know what they can't do. They already focus on what they can't do. Feedback is about figuring out what you can do.*
>
> —*Cheryl Weinstein, Ph.D.*

Helping patients develop a long-term plan

Patients may feel overwhelmed by too many recommendations, especially when clinicians may be anxious to try to fit everything in because there might not be an opportunity to see them again. An alternative to long lists of recommendations is to map out a five-year plan, and then have regular check-ins to follow up. It's harder in this insurance environment to see people back in person, but you can do it with emails. The goal is to set up a back-and-forth collaboration.

> o *(This concept of discussing five-year plans comes from Jane Bernstein.) "These are your strengths, and these are your weaknesses—this is what gets in the way. Let's plot out what will happen in the next five years. This is what you can first tackle. If it works, then this is what you can look forward to working on next. If it doesn't work, and you get off track, let's figure out how to get back on track. Let us know what's working or not working; we can follow up with emails."*
>
> —*Cheryl Weinstein, Ph.D.*

Creating opportunities for success

Sometimes a child has been unable to succeed because they have not been placed in a setting that is appropriate for their unique set of needs, and constant failing leads to a sense of learned helplessness. Sometimes it's not the school's fault, it's not the kid's fault, it's not the parent's fault—the team has just not yet found the right fit for the child to help foster success.

> o *Kids don't generally fail in all settings. They don't tend to succeed in all settings. The goal is to try to maximize those settings where they succeed and determine how we can foster this. There is an effect of chronically feeling like you've failed: learned helplessness is a real thing. But learned efficacy is also a real thing. If you believe that you succeed, you tend to succeed at things more: Success fosters success.*
>
> —*Keith Owen Yeates, Ph.D.*

Road map metaphor for encouraging compensatory strategies

o *"Before the injury/illness, you knew your way around perfectly. You took freeways, and got straight from point A to point B directly—no problem. Now, you have to learn different ways of getting there—or you may need a map to get there. You need some aids. Now, rather than going straight from point A to B, you may need to take some side streets. You'll still get there, but it might take longer. And you may need to stop and get directions on the way."*

—Munro Cullum, Ph.D.

Bunion metaphor for executive dysfunction compensatory strategies

o *Bunions, similar to executive vulnerabilities, are annoying, chronic conditions which respond well to accommodations. Both also require continual monitoring. For example, if you stress the bunion by wearing the wrong shoe, the bunion becomes painful and walking is difficult. Because some people love beautiful, but uncomfortable shoes, the bunion becomes irritated and walking/movement is severely curtailed. To walk without pain, selecting a different shoe is necessary. However, the underlying condition never goes away.*

It is the same with executive dysfunction. Individuals use strategies that improve executive functioning, such as planning the next day. Life becomes easier. As time passes, planning ahead may seem repetitive and boring … just like wearing the comfortable, but boring shoe. If planning stops, things can feel overwhelming again. When planning and making accommodations resume, things get better. Just like bunions. Over time, using these compensatory strategies will become less cumbersome, but its usefulness will not diminish.

—Winifred Hentschel, Ed.D.

Encouraging patience in finding the right compensatory strategies

A lot of parents want you to define for them what their kids can and cannot do, but the reality is that we cannot always do that without any trial and error.

o *"You will have to test the waters and see what they can and cannot do. You will have to be more flexible, and let things be dynamic."*

—Jim Scott, Ph.D.

Talking with patients about alternative treatments

This is a good way to talk to patients about treatments that are not evidence-based (e.g., hyperbaric oxygen, interactive metronome, and diets, if they are innocuous.)

o *"I can tell you this, I don't necessarily think it's going to hurt you (your child), but I haven't seen evidence yet that it makes a big difference. It costs a lot of money and it's not covered by your insurance. If I thought that it really made a difference I would tell you, but I have not seen studies that says it does. There are people who will try to sell you things. You may go on a website and see testimonials—some are paid. But testimonials are different from large, well-designed studies."*

—*Jacobus Donders, Ph.D.*

INTRODUCING COMPENSATORY STRATEGIES FOR MEMORY

These techniques are helpful ways to introduce compensatory strategies for memory problems across many patient types and syndromes.

o *It is very helpful for patients when clinicians normalize the need for organizational/ memory compensatory strategies. I use myself as an example." (My office is a mess—books open, papers on the table. ...)*

"Look at how chaotic my life is. The only reason I can get things done is because I keep a checklist of all the things I need to do. Every morning when I come in, I check to see what I need to do. If you learn to compensate, you can lead an independent life. If you don't compensate, then the memory problems could take over to the point where you can't live independently. You can take charge."

—*John Lucas, Ph.D.*

o *"I can never remember my husband's relatives' names. So we do cue cards before we go to a wedding—with names, and little notes about family members." (I pull out my notebook). "Look, this is about who's got to be where. What I have to do, what I need to say to people. It's all in there. You can do this too. You are going to get the most gorgeous daily planner so you can say, 'I'm important.' And you are going to look at it three times a day, at 8:00, 12:00, and 6:00. You will come back in a month and tell me how this works—what is working, and what is not working. We will then make changes that work for you."*

—*Cheryl Weinstein, Ph.D.*

Simple solutions for memory support

o *Sometimes it's really simple. Sometimes it's just like developing good mental habits to relieve the burden on the memory system—like maybe just always putting your car keys in the same place.*

—*Gordon Chelune, Ph.D.*

Four techniques to support memory

When I discuss memory strategies, I emphasize four different issues: organization, repetition, elaboration, and attitude.

o **Organization**—"*When trying to remember information from a conversation, you should become an active participant and elaborate, reflect, question, and reframe what the speaker is saying. This will turn a monologue into a dialogue, which makes the speaker slow down and which gives you a second pass at information.*" (*And then we practice it.*)

Repetition—"*Your brain responds to novelty. So, your job is to use novelty when you repeat information. You might repeat something in a different way or at a different time. Repeating information in different ways capitalizes on the novelty effect and it also enhances the network or contacts of each memory, making them stronger.*"

Or: "*Part of your brain that is very involved in memory is your hippocampus. Your hippocampus gets bored by repeated information and falls asleep. If I put electrodes on your brain and said my name three times in a row, your hippocampus would fall asleep. So, your job is to use novelty when you repeat. The way you get novelty is either by repeating something in a different way or by repeating it at a different time. Repetition is key, but it's the way you repeat it that's even more important. Novelty also makes different contacts, so it's organized different ways conceptually.*"

Elaboration—"*Elaboration helps you to remember information that might otherwise be tricky to retain. For instance, if my name is Jill Smith, you might think of someone you knew in fifth grade named Smith. When you do this, you establish different addresses that are useful when it's time to look up information.*"

Attitude—"*The most important tool is your attitude. It is important to figure out what you will say in situations when you have a memory lapse. You may not want to say that you are having a 'senior moment,' because that's self-effacing. You might say something more assertive such as 'I'm blocking on your name.' Even 20-year-olds refer to 'blocking.'*" (*I encourage people to develop their own personal mantra to get off the hook when they're having a memory lapse*).

—*Margaret O'Connor, Ph.D.*

RECOMMENDING PSYCHOTHERAPY

With a patient who is really depressed—the most important thing is safety. Feedback becomes a therapeutic session. I use this approach as one doorway to that conversation:

o "*The good news is your brain is functioning just fine, but I'm really worried about you.*"

—*Robin Hilsabeck, Ph.D.*

o "*When I'm talking about counseling and psychotherapy—I'm not talking about lying on the couch and crying about your mother. I'm talking about how do you get through your day, given all this stress you are dealing with? I am going to send you to someone who can talk with you about coping, not crying over spilt milk."*

—*Jacobus Donders, Ph.D.*

○ *I give patients an example, "You're taking a test and can't answer a question. Then you have this, 'Oh my god!' response and become anxious and can't continue. CBT helps you identify this moment, challenge the thought, and change it, so you can take the tests more easily."*

—*Robb Mapou, Ph.D.*

The following strategy avoids an argument or struggle about whether the patient should go to psychotherapy. Patients are just listening to your "wonderings."

○ *"It seems like you're going through a really hard time. What would you think about getting treatment for depression? I wonder what that would be like? Do you think that might help with being able to take your meds? I wonder if it would help with these problems we've just talked about with the way your brain is working?"*

—*Monica Mindt, Ph.D.*

PEARLS TO FACILITATE CONNECTING WITH DIVERSE CULTURES

Cultural knowledge gives you an estimate, but you still have to find out whether it applies to a particular individual. I use this pearl for Italian patients. They can tell I am Chinese. If they respond to that, then that tells me, okay, family issues are very important. This leads me to other hypotheses ... more traditional, Old World culture. They may treat emotional issues in a more traditional way. It tells me to tread lightly.

○ *"I love my Italian patients. You all are very family-oriented. I find that we have this in common. And we like pasta—we like noodles and are family-oriented."*
—*Tony Wong, Ph.D.*

To sit down with someone from Alaskan Native culture and begin asking him or her about alcohol abuse in the family—how rude can you get? In general, Alaskan Natives will be quiet until they feel comfortable. They do not feel comfortable jumping right in and sharing personal information. When giving feedback, it is important that the way I am communicating be understandable and culturally appropriate. There is a slower pace of conversation expected in Alaskan Native culture. To acknowledge I am being rude by asking so many questions can be disarming. Most Alaskan Natives typically say, "Okay." The following can be said at the initial evaluation session, as well as during feedback sessions, particularly as family members may be present who were not able to attend the first meeting.

o *"If I were meeting you socially, I would not be so nosy. I would like to apologize for being so nosy—but it's my job, and I want to do it well."*

—Paul Craig, Ph.D.

Discussing lack of norms for diverse populations

Discussing the lack of neuropsychological norms for a patient's culture is important both during the consent phase of the initial consultation and during feedback.

o *"Unfortunately I don't have any tests that were specifically developed and normed among Alaskan Natives. I realize that there is cultural bias inherent to the test and I take that into consideration when interpreting the test. So your score as shown in this report on the verbal scale is in the low-average range, but that is driven by the cultural bias associated with the items contained in that test. Compared with your cultural cohort—the people within your community—you are very normal. On this naming test and on the vocabulary test, I know and you know—there are a lot of words we could put on the test that you would know and that people from New York would not."*

—Paul Craig, Ph.D.

o *"The way we understand whether a test score is normal is we compare your score to the scores of a group of people like you. And by 'you,' I mean the same age and even the same ethnicity. Mr. C, as a field right now, we don't have good normative data for people similar to you. So the best way to see what's going on for you is to do more than one set of tests. Then I can compare your scores to someone exactly like you—I can compare you directly to yourself—how you do now, versus six months from now."*

—Desiree White, Ph.D.

o *"I would prefer to be camping with you, than some guy from New York who has a high score on this test. These tests don't measure everything important in your culture. It tends to measure things important in the culture it was created in. You know how to survive in the bush. People from New York know how to survive in a very different environment."*

—Paul Craig, Ph.D.

INTRODUCING RELIGIOUS IDEAS

When appropriate in the context of patients' expressed beliefs, introducing religious concepts can be a powerful tool for feedback. The initial clinical interview is a good time to gauge the extent and content of patients' religious beliefs. If interview data suggest that religion is an important part of a patient's emotional support system, then this information can be utilized in the feedback session.

o *In the interview I might say something like: "You've told me about these problems you've had. You told me you don't have thoughts of suicide. I'm glad you don't, but what holds you up?" Then in the feedback session, depending on how they are reacting to the news: Anger? Despair? "How can you enjoy the time that the Lord has given you… ?" (If sitting there with a WWJD bracelet): "What do you think Jesus would want you to do?"*

—*Jacobus Donders, Ph.D.*

OFFERING FEEDBACK TO PILOTS

Regardless of the neurological issue that triggered the assessment, this pearl helps introduce test results in pilot evaluations: ultimately, the Federal Aviation Administration (FAA) makes final decisions.

○ *"Neuropsychological testing is not an assessment of aviation skills. It's an assessment of how you are able to perform on these tasks that have been demonstrated to be sensitive to brain functions. With regard to these tests, they have been normed against a population of commercial pilots. I have results against which to compare you—to your peers—on these particular tasks. My gold standard with regard to aviation based upon what I know about you neuropsychologically, is—would I get in a plane with you flying? If the answer is no, I need to communicate that in my report. I realize the test results do not tell me anything about your competence as an aviator. Rather, the tests tell me how you perform on tasks specific to brain function compared with other pilots."*

—*Paul Craig, Ph.D.*

○ *"Mr. Smith, I know you think you can fly the plane. But we performed the set of tests the FAA requested, and you had significant problems with memory, attention, and problem solving. I hear you when you say that you can use pre-flight checklists, just like you have done for 30 years. But you have to remember, I am not making this decision, the medical director at the FAA is making the decision. And really, the FAA medical director isn't making the decision either. He is bound by a set of government regulations. If you fail the tests, he can't let you fly. And you know government regulations from your days in the military! I know you think you can manage, and you are very charming—but it's not about making a great argument to me or to the FAA. It's the government—and their regulations. If you fail the tests, they have to go by the book."*

—*Karen Postal, Ph.D.*

GENERAL PEARLS FOR THE PEDIATRIC POPULATION

Joining with parents when explaining recommendations

○ *If the context is appropriate, I may say, "I try to look at your child not just as a neuropsychologist, but as a mother. If she were my child, what would I do? So I'll tell you, if it was my child, I would.…"*

—*Cynthia Levinson, Ph.D.*

Case manager metaphor for parental role

Family members can be empowered by identifying their role in supporting the patient.

o *"I am the professional in the evaluation, but you are the case manager."*
—*Rebecca Wilson, Psy.D.*

Dinner vs. Cafeteria metaphor for program planning

Here is a great rationale for home-schooling or placing kids with autistic spectrum disorder in a specialized academic environment or school. This metaphor is also helpful for talking with kids in high school and helping them look forward to college.

o *"Regular school is like a family dinner. You get whatever mom serves. They make you do something specific. And it doesn't work for everybody. Life is like a cafeteria. 'I like that, not that, and I will have the chocolate pudding.' You may be a good skier and I might be a good golfer, because we are better at some things than others. Brown University doesn't have any required courses at all. That's the way real life is. I can do what I want to do. If it doesn't pay off, I may have to conform my behavior a bit more, but I have a lot of choices in how much payoff I am looking for, and how much conformity I accept. Let's try to get to 'the cafeteria' for Jack. Let's find kids who are like him now, rather than wait till he's an adult." (Or "Let's find an educational environment he can survive in now. Let's not wait 18 years.") "Let's just do it right now."*
—*Tom Boll, Ph.D.*

Standard transmission metaphor for children with special needs

This is a useful metaphor for any child with developmental or learning disabilities or autistic spectrum disorder.

o *"Average kids, they're like a car with an automatic transmission. You put your foot on the gas, and everything takes care of itself. You send them to school, and 12 years later they graduate. Your kid has a standard"* (stick shift) *"transmission. Any time you want him to learn something, you have to remember that you need to give explicit instructions. 'You move your left leg, and your right arm, and then move your left leg, and move your arm....' There's a whole series of things you need to teach him/tell him that are very specific. Your son is a standard-transmission kid. You can't just put him in the car and have him step on the gas. If you just put him in the car and hope everything works—it won't. You will always have to remember that you need to teach him to shift."[Tailor this to the specific disorder; e.g., autism spectrum. For example, "If you want him to understand kids, you will have to explicitly train him with social skills training, just like algebra training. It won't just come naturally"].*
—*Tom Boll, Ph.D.*

Recalibrating parents' visions for children with acquired cognitive deficits

After an acute illness is over, families need to recalibrate their vision for their child. This applies to developmental disabilities as well as acute illness. The message to families is that it doesn't matter what their child's cognitive abilities are, they still have to try. They may have to adjust their goals, but children still have to try hard to do whatever they are going to do.

○ *"Keep challenging Debbie. Even though she was sick, it doesn't mean she gets to stop trying. It's just like everyone else, whether you had a life-threatening illness or not. You have to try. That's how success is measured, not by achievement, but by effort."*

—*Jim Scott, Ph.D.*

Encouraging interventions, even when parents are not ready to accept diagnoses

Some parents react to feedback by providing alternative explanations for low scores (e.g., "Oh, she gets really shy around people"). In these instances, it is helpful to differentiate between risk factors and skill deficits.

○ *"Your daughter is still young, and what we are seeing may still be separation issues, or shyness around strangers" (join with the parents' hypothesis). "What I am concerned about is, if this is the way she continues to be, and we don't work on developing those social skills, that when she is in kindergarten for six hours a day, she will be at high risk. So why don't we think of this as a risk factor for social skill problems, rather than a social skill deficit? It makes a lot of sense to intervene now, before it becomes a deficit."*

—*Jennifer Turek Queally, Ph.D.*

Discussing developmental trajectories

○ *"The child has a developmental trajectory, but so does the family—Mom gets a job when the third child goes to school; the older sister goes to college; the grandfather moves in with the family after grandmother dies. We're just looking at one frame in Jill's development. And childhood is a movie."*

—*Christopher J. Nicholls, Ph.D.*

This is one way to help parents understand that their expectations might not be in line with their child's developmental stage:

○ *"One day, the child just clicks in to the next stage, like puberty. And if you are expecting your child to be performing at a higher stage, it can be really frustrating. I see a lot of children who suddenly 'get' organization of homework, or another task that they have been asked 100 times to do. And it's not because they were asked 101 times, it's because they are now at the next developmental stage."*

—*Molly Warner, Ph.D.*

Establishing realistic expectations

Sometimes the most important intervention to get across to parents is to, in effect, tell the parent to back off—in a nice way.

o *"Actually, your kid's okay. They're not going to be a Harvard scholar. Get used to that, but recognize and celebrate what they are."*
— *Keith Owen Yeates, Ph.D.*

Framing a parent's disability as a positive model for their child

Parents may present with social skills deficits very similar to their child's. They may also have dyslexia or attention deficits. These may have been previously acknowledged in the family, but sometimes the assessment is the first time that the parents' own developmental difference has been acknowledged. This can be framed positively:

o *"You are a unique and wonderful resource for your child."*
— *Rebecca Wilson, Psy.D.*

PARTING WORDS

Calming a catastrophic reaction

Some people are devastated upon hearing the neuropsychological feedback. As a neuropsychologist, one never wants to do any emotional harm. Physicians do no physical harm. Neuropsychologists should do no emotional harm with feedback, but this can be challenging to do at times. This pearl reminds patients that the *diagnosis* (or other feedback) does not change the person:

o *"You are the same person as when you walked in here. You can do the same things. You can take your vacation. Go out to dinner."*
— *Sara J. Swanson, Ph.D.*

6   Dementia

FEEDBACK SESSIONS INVOLVING Alzheimer disease and related dementia syndromes may be particularly challenging due to a patient's lack of awareness, complex and changing family dynamics involved in caregiving, and significant safety issues. This chapter provides pearls that address all of these topics as well as ways to encourage caregivers to take care of themselves.

DISCUSSING DEMENTIA AND MEMORY LOSS WITH FAMILIES AND PATIENTS

Providing an initial diagnosis relating to memory problems and dementia typically involves educating patients and their family members about the differences between the normal effects of aging, mild cognitive impairment (MCI), and various stages of dementia.

Explaining the continuum of memory function

o *"One of the reasons you came to see me is that you or a family member noticed that there has been a decline in your memory. There's a long list of factors that can affect memory in someone your age, including just the effects of normal aging. So there's a continuum here from perfectly normal memory function all the way to a patient lying in a nursing home with severe dementia. We go from perfect cognitive function, to normal cognitive function for one's age. One of our first determinations is, do we think there is a decline in memory function beyond what we would account for by effects of normal aging? And if so, what is the effect on your normal daily activity? There is a category of mild cognitive impairment—this person has more changes in cognitive function beyond what could be accounted for by normal aging, but not sufficient to call it dementia. And beyond that, does this warrant the category of dementia? If so, what stage is it—is it mild, moderate or severe?*

In your case, my concern is that we are beyond the effects of normal aging. You and your husband are telling me that there is a significant impact on your ability to drive and balance the checkbook, and it's having an effect on your normal activities. My concern here is that we're in the early stages of a dementia. And if that is the case, what is the likely cause? There are various types of dementia. We need to use clinical characteristics and test results to tell what type of dementia you have and how to treat it."

—*Michael McCrea, Ph.D.*

Distinguishing between normal aging and memory loss

Due to unawareness, many patients hearing they have a severe memory deficit will say, "But all my friends have memory problems too," or "Yes, I know I have some memory problems. It's just aging." The following method of introducing memory results is helpful in short-circuiting this process.

o *"Mrs. Smith, last week you came in and did a bunch of memory tests. We give those tests to thousands of people your age. So we can compare your memory directly to others who are also 80. And even though you still have your smarts, you have a really severe memory problem. Compared to a typical 80-year-old, your intellect is up here (hand high in the air) but your memory is way down here (hand low). So this isn't just the effect of normal aging. What we are looking at is a memory problem that is worse than just normal aging."*

—*Karen Postal, Ph.D.*

Addressing a family's alternative explanations for memory loss

At times it is clear that family members or caregivers are very highly invested in memory problems' being something other than Alzheimer disease. They might be clinging to the idea that a concussion five years ago was the cause of their mother's memory problems, or that grief for a spouse who passed a few years ago is causing all of the functional difficulties. As clinicians, one of our roles is to bring in reality. Family members can't help the patient if they don't understand the extent of their problems. Even when they are saying it is due to something else, they likely have a significant fear that the cause is a degenerative dementia. The following conversation gives them permission to discuss the "elephant in the room":

o *"You can get the flu and break your arm. It's possible that there's more than one thing contributing to a situation. We've found significant memory problems here. What are you concerned might be the cause other than grieving?"*

—*John Lucas, Ph.D.*

Reassuring patients with memory loss about preserved skills

Some people feel dumb when they are given a dementia diagnosis. It is important to talk up their strengths to help *avoid* this reaction.

o *"You're just as bright as ever. Some things my have changed, but for example, your vocabulary is where it was, and that's a strength."*

—*Munro Cullum, Ph.D.*

MILD COGNITIVE IMPAIRMENT

Explaining mild cognitive impairment in a manner that accurately captures the significance of the cognitive changes, while not creating excessive anxiety in patients and families, is an art.

Explaining MCI

o *"You can't have dementia if you can do all of your everyday tasks independently. So let me tell you right now, you don't have dementia. But your memory really isn't where it should be. And we'll have to watch it."* (Maybe the patient will get Alzheimer disease, but right now, she's not demented, and she does not need to feel like she is being punched in the face with a diagnosis.)

—*Sara J. Swanson, Ph.D.*

How mild cognitive impairment is presented in feedback often depends on the clinicians' level of suspicion about the trajectory the cognitive changes are likely to take.

○ *"This is a border zone between normal aging and dementia. This is not dementia at this point. Some folks stay with this level of memory impairment for years. Others will progress—about 10 percent of people per year do get worse."* (Emphasize one course or another based on test results. If it looks like AD, say:) *"Many times this progresses and gets worse. We don't know who will end up progressing. I can't tell you in three years how you will be doing, but I do recommend that you be followed annually, or earlier than that if you see major changes."*

—*Munro Cullum, Ph.D.*

When cognitive differences are subtle enough for a low suspicion of an early dementia, clinicians can leave the door open for patients to return while at the same time reassuring them that conversion to dementia is unlikely.

○ *"You know, this is a good baseline. If you see anything in a year, you can come back and we will retest. But I'd be surprised if you're back."*

—*Richard Naugle, Ph.D.*

Waiting room metaphor for mci

○ *"You're not in the area of dementia, but you're not in the normal area. It's like you're in the waiting room of memory. We aren't sure what will happen. We are going to watch you closely over the next year. When we re-evaluate you, we will then have two points to make a line. Up, down, or straight."* (Draw in the air with your hands).

—*Bill Barr, Ph.D.*

Yellow light metaphor for MCI

○ *"We're seeing a few problems here, but they're not severe. So it's a yellow-light situation; we need to proceed with caution. We'll re-evaluate again later and keep track of how things are going."*

—*John Randolph, Ph.D.*

Radar metaphor for mci

This is a great metaphor for the post–World War II crowd.

○ *"We're seeing a few blips on the radar here. We don't know clearly what they are, but we're going to track them."*

—*John J. Randolph, Ph.D.*

Validating patient's decision to be tested when scores are normal

Some patients feel embarrassed when memory testing turns out to be normal. On these occasions it is important to reassure them that their decision to come for testing was sound.

> o *"It may be that you sat through three hours of testing, and we didn't find anything. But you didn't waste your time. We have a good baseline here."*
>
> —*Richard Naugle, Ph.D.*

USING THE "A" WORD—ALZHEIMER DISEASE

Clinicians vary in their use of the words "Alzheimer disease" with patients and families. Some intentionally avoid using the term, or use it only when specifically asked the name of the dementia by a patient or family member. Other clinicians regularly use the term, feeling that patients and their families have come to them for a clear diagnosis and might be misled if the diagnosis is not used. Whatever the ultimate strategy, the use of the word "Alzheimer" can be highly charged, and deciding when to use it warrants thoughtful preparation.

In my experience, you don't need to use the "A-word." With early Alzheimer disease, we can't offer definitive disease-modifying therapy. So telling a patient directly that it's Alzheimer can be more frightening than telling them they have cancer. The earlier in the disease process the diagnosis is made, the more likely the patient is to understand the implications of what it means to have Alzheimer. They might have a full-blown emotional response that perhaps you didn't need to evoke.

On the other hand, there are some patients who come right out and say, "I want to know." They may want to make plans—put their life in order, cross off as many items on their bucket list as they can. You know, buy the sports car, take the around-the-world trip. They want to know so they can do it now. In those cases I will be more blunt.

In these limited instances, people ask directly. But generally patients need to harbor some hope, some sense that by the dint of their efforts they might be able to make a difference in the ultimate outcome. I don't think that it's our job to take a sledgehammer to someone's denial.

> o *"There are really no surprises here. You were concerned about your memory. Indeed, the examination gives good reasons for that. I have serious concerns for your memory at this point. I think you have a problem, which I don't think will get any better. In fact I suspect it will continue to get worse. There's always a chance I could be wrong. But I have a lot of confidence in what I am saying to you."*
>
> —*Aaron Nelson, Ph.D.*

On the other hand, many practitioners feel that the using the word "Alzheimer" is important for clarity and treatment planning.

> o *"If I had Stage 4 carcinoma, and a very low chance of survival, would you tell me? Yes, because I need to get my affairs in order. So do patients with Alzheimer's disease."*
>
> —*Susan McPherson, Ph.D.*

Sometimes a patient's child or children call before a scheduled feedback session and ask to hear the assessment results prior to the family meeting. Often, their purpose is to protect their parent from hearing the word "Alzheimer." In some situations, such as when a daughter disclosed that her father had always said he would kill himself if he had the disease, I might agree to using a euphemism such as, "the type of memory problem that gets worse over time." Typically, though, I discuss the benefits of naming the problem, and reassure the family member that the patient's emotional response is often not as catastrophic as they fear.

o *"Even though you all have suspected something was going on for a few years, hearing the words 'Alzheimer disease' can be very jarring and upsetting. "I was involved in a research project a few years back, looking at the effect on patients of hearing the word 'Alzheimer.' It turns out, that while the family members were very, appropriately upset by the word, the use of the term actually had very little impact on patients. Typically they did not recall the diagnosis even a few days later. One of the changes that occurs early in the dementia process is a dulling and disconnecting of emotions. Many patients, when they hear the word 'Alzheimer,' have mild reactions, or even very little reaction at all, something that would be unthinkable for them prior to the disease.*

"Mostly, because of the lack of awareness that goes along with Alzheimer's, patients just think you are wrong. The part of their brain that could know they were having memory problems—that part is broken. This is one of the reasons, though, that frankly discussing the diagnosis can be important. Being able to reference this conversation—'Mom, do you remember when we met with Dr. Postal, she said that because you have Alzheimer disease, a really bad memory problem, I need to be the one to count out your pills in the pill box each week?' Being able to go back to this discussion is very helpful."

—Karen Postal, Ph.D.

Patients and family know something is not right. Feedback is the time to name it. Finding a gentle way to introduce the word can be challenging, but it often can be facilitated by offering information about what to do next.

Family members can be very anxious about delivering a diagnosis to the patient. Some people are prepared for it. Some are not even remotely prepared. I always meander to the word "Alzheimer." I often say "Alzheimer-like." I don't have a slide with plaques and tangles. I like to allow a softer landing, while giving the bad news.

o *"This is the sort of problem we see in patients with Alzheimer disease." (Fodder for discussion. People say anything from "Holy %$#!" to "We suspected that was the case.")*

—Greg Lamberty, Ph.D.

o *"This is more than normal aging. There's something wrong with your brain. It's most likely Alzheimer's. Regardless of the label we put on it, let's talk about what we are going to do about it."*

—Jacobus Donders, Ph.D.

Labeling the diagnosis can be empowering

o *"Knowledge about dementia can be painful. But it will allow you, when you are ready, to make the best decisions to maintain your mother's quality of life.... Knowledge can also be power."*

—Cynthia Kubu, Ph.D.

Calla lily metaphor for alzheimer's disease

o *"The word we're going to use might be Alzheimer's disease, but for the sake of argument, let's call it 'calla lily.' It's much prettier. It doesn't change what it is. But it's a lot prettier. Let's call your problem 'calla lily.' Let's talk about what this is.... Now we're going to talk about how we treat calla lily, and how we keep calla lily beautiful as long as possible. Water and food keep the system intact as long as possible. We don't want you to get an infection, because that will hurt the system. We can also use cholinesterase medication to keep it healthy as long as possible. We want to help keep it as long as possible, because we know no plant goes along forever."*

—Mark Barisa, Ph.D.

CAREGIVER ISSUES

Alzheimer's and other dementia patients often have poor awareness of their deficits, and feel physically well. They may not feel like patients in need of intervention. In those situations, families hold the understanding of the illness and have the burden of caring for an individual who neither knows they need care nor welcomes intervention. During feedback sessions, therefore, many messages spoken to patients are primarily directed towards educating their spouses and children about caregiving issues. These range from discussions relating to physical and financial safety, to planning for late-stage care, to handling the emotional burdens of caregiving.

HELPING CAREGIVERS UNDERSTAND AND MANAGE THEIR LOVED ONE'S DEFICITS

Caregivers can become very frustrated with demented family members. For example, they may complain about what appears to be "selective memory." That is, the patient only forgets what is "convenient." They can also become annoyed by repetitive questions, conversations, and behaviors. Feedback sessions are a prime opportunity to help caregivers better understand the disease process, as well as to develop an awareness of what it is like to be in the patient's shoes, living moment by moment.

o *"It's not uncommon at all to be able to remember things better from their past. Memory loss proceeds backwards, so your mom should be able to talk about her past. At times, she may actually believe she is in her past."*

—Julie Keaveney, Psy.D.

o *"Your mother's memory is such that she probably feels like at any given time she is in a completely unfamiliar kind of circumstance. She doesn't remember what was just said. She doesn't know how to participate in the conversation, because how can I know what to say in a conversation when I don't know what was just said? She doesn't remember why she is there or what she is supposed to be doing. And there's a lot of anxiety in that situation—not knowing. So when she asks you to repeat things, in that moment, you need to believe that she really needs to know."*

—Julie Keaveney, Psy.D.

Incontinence and dementia

Incontinence can be a significant problem for families. Often they do not understand its source, and they become increasingly frustrated. Explaining *why* the patient is having toileting difficulties can be instrumental in helping families to cope more effectively with the problem.

o *"It's really an issue of your husband's neurological condition. He is not trying to wet the bed—or be incontinent. It's part of his dementia. He may be forgetting to go to the bathroom, or not be aware of the growing need. I know it's tough. It's not a willful thing—it is part of the neurological condition. It's important to not be frustrated/angry with the person."*

—Robin Hanks, Ph.D.

Explaining mismatch between caregiver communication style and patient deficits

Many family members become very frustrated by caregiving activities and daily interactions with their spouse or parent who has dementia. A mismatch between old styles of communication that worked well for decades, and the patient's current cognitive abilities may be part of the problem. For example, a fast-paced delivery of a message, or an expectation that the patient will be able to hold more than one thing in mind at a time, may lead to frequent miscommunications.

o *"Do you have a sense that how you communicate with your loved one helps or doesn't help? Are you talking too quickly? Slow down. Slow down while speaking and slow down with what you do. Make sure you allow for a lot of extra time to get ready. Also, do you think you might be talking too much? Sometimes it helps to say less.*

Do you tend to point out his mistakes? Nobody likes to be told they are wrong, and sometimes this can fuel frustration. If he makes a mistake, try ignoring it and ask yourself, 'does it really matter if he thinks it's Tuesday but it's not?' You can also try to make it seem as though it was actually your mistake, and apologize. For example, you can tell him, 'Oh, I'm sorry, I forgot to tell you!'

"Is there one person who can get the patient to do almost anything? It may be helpful to look at what that person does, and see how it differs from those who seem to struggle more with him."

—Tanis Ferman, Ph.D.

Mirroring in neurodegenerative dementia

o *"Are you finding that if you are in a bad mood, he's in a bad mood? If you are calm, he is calm? If you are aggravated, does she seem more irritable? Do his moods mirror your moods? With some neurological changes to the brain, something called 'mirroring' occurs where your loved one may mimic your moods."*

—Tanis Ferman, Ph.D.

"Don't tell Dad Mom's dead again:" avoiding repeated traumatizing in dementia

Family members often feel they need to correct a patient's memory mistakes or they will worsen. One of the worst mistakes is correcting them when they discuss a close loved on as if they were still alive, because doing so in essence is breaking the traumatic news of a loved one's death.

o *"At some point it's possible that your mother will forget some major fact, like that a loved one or spouse has died. Remember, from their perspective they have no memory of that. So when they ask, 'Where's dad, I haven't seen him lately, he must be working really hard,' that's their reality. When you say, 'Mom, don't you remember that dad died five years ago!?' it is like you are giving [her] this horrible news for the first time; it is very upsetting or bewildering! And then they will forget. How many times are you going to give this traumatic news? The better plan if this happens is to divert and deflect—'Oh, he's fine,' and change the topic, because they will forget what they were talking about and then you avoid the emotional trauma. If the person flat-out asks you, 'Did he die?' I don't advise you to lie. If they have a direct question, you can tell them, but you don't need to offer."*

If the family says, "do you want me to lie?" I tell them, "If your family member was totally rational, able to benefit from new information, think it through, and evaluate it, then yes, you would be lying to them, because you're giving them no opportunity to reconcile the information on their own. But that's not the case. Your family member has a 30-second to one-minute memory window, and it is counterproductive to tell them things that are upsetting only to have to tell them over and over again."

—Julie Keaveney, Psy.D.

Encouraging caregivers to take care of themselves—and to share the burden among family members

o *"Caregiving is often a challenge to people. Are you taking care of yourself? What do you do to get out of the situation? What are your outside activities and hobbies? You need to think about, 'What if something happens to me?' You need to make sure that you get a chance to exercise, go out. You need to give yourself permission to do this. This is part of your job as a caregiver: to take care of yourself. If you are in good health emotionally and physically, then you can take the best care of your spouse."*

—Munro Cullum, Ph.D.

○ *"Your ability to care for your spouse is going to be dependant on your ability to care for yourself. You need to make sure your needs are balanced with the caregiving demands." (To patients)—"One of the greatest gifts that anyone gives to another person is to allow that person to help them. When you help another person you feel good about yourself. That is the great gift you give to them. Was there ever a time when you helped someone else—and did you feel good about yourself? I have a feeling that may be the way your family member or spouse feels about caring for you." (To spouse)—"Is that how you feel?" (They usually say yes). (Turning back to the spouse)—"But it's also time-consuming, and takes a lot of energy. So we want to make sure you get the benefits of both— caregiving, and also taking care of yourself so you have the ability to do this great job."*

—*Robin Hanks, Ph.D.*

In most instances, caregiving is not a one-person job, and it helps to have some respite. Some caregivers perceive seeking help as a personal failure. In such circumstances, enlisting the caregiver's willingness to obtain help may require a clear understanding of what they feel would really be *useful*; we must never assume that we know what is best for a particular caregiver. Sometimes when it is put in the context of what the patient needs, a caregiver may be willing to obtain extra help.

○ *"It doesn't matter how old or young you are, caregiving is never a one-person job. Take a look at your situation and ask, 'What kind of help do we need?' Some folks need help with bathing and dressing, others need somebody to do the housework and some cooking, others need a driver, and others need a nighttime sitter. If you can get into a routine, where your helper comes in the same times and days each week, then both you and your husband will know what to expect and it may make things easier. Sometimes a day program or a daytime companion gives your loved one more structure and contact with others, and gives you a much needed break."*

—*Tanis Ferman, Ph.D.*

○ *"You must take care of yourself. That is not selfish. The exercise is your time. You deserve it. Two days you exercise by yourself, maybe the third and fourth time you can do something with your family. Walks, skiing, there's got to be something."*

—*Cheryl Weinstein, Ph.D.*

○ *"Let's just pretend that I don't care about you at all. The only person I care about is the patient. I would still tell you that you've got to get help. That you've got to get relief; that you've got to get support. Not because I like you, because we've agreed I don't like you at all, but because if you collapse the whole thing goes down. And the patient that I care about dissolves, because he needs you. So it's not because I'm being nice to you or because I want you to feel selfish, it's because the system needs you and without you it collapses."*

—*Tom Boll, Ph.D.*

Marathon metaphor for caregiving

o *"Caring for someone with Alzheimer's is like running a marathon, not a sprint. You need to make sure that you refuel yourself along the way, and conserve energy."*
—*Cynthia Kubu, Ph.D.*

Airplane emergency oxygen metaphor for caregiving

o *"Right before your airplane takes off, do you know how flight attendants tell you to put the oxygen mask on yourself first, before you put it on your child? It's really startling to hear that. Can you imagine not helping your own child first when the plane is going down? But it makes sense, when you think it through. Because if you have passed out from lack of oxygen, how are you going to help your child survive? Mrs. Smith, if you don't start taking care of yourself, how will you make it long enough to care for your husband? He's going to need you. If you want to care for him, you have to care for yourself as well."*
—*Karen Postal, Ph.D.*

Supporting caregivers with family conflict

Sometimes family members feel that they need to resolve old issues (e.g., abusive relationships) before they can be caregivers. Unfortunately, there are times when a patient is simply no longer capable of such a discussion.

o *"That ship has sailed. This person is no longer that person. He no longer has the capacity to understand what happened in the past. If you have things to say to your dad that you haven't before, now is not the time. That time has passed. It won't make any impact."*
—*Laurie Ryan, Ph.D.*

Facilitating family cooperation in caregiving

o *"I think in the next few days, it will be time to have a family pow-wow. Get every-one around a table and say we have these needs: 'Dad can't drive anymore, some-one needs to grocery shop. How we are going to divvy up the pie?'"*
—*Michael McCrea, Ph.D.*

In some situations the family members who are furthest away geographically may deny the severity of the patient's dementia. This forces the family members who are closer to the patient to caregive without assistance.

o *"No, he's not fine. He has dementia, and your sister's dying on the vine here. She needs some help. When it all falls on one person it's a recipe for disaster—not only for your dad, who needs the care. It's a disaster for the one who is carrying all the heavy bags."*
—*Michael McCrea, Ph.D.*

Facilitating family cooperation in caregiving: get your brothers off their behinds

Daughters and daughters-in-law tend to be stuck with a disproportionate share of caregiving. This leads to burnout, and ultimately worse care for patients.

o *"You know, caregiving burdens tend to fall on the women in the family. So get your brothers off their behinds and involved in the care." (If brothers are in the room)—"If this is all going to fall on one or two people, you will have a disaster on your hands, because that person is going to burn out quickly. So, everybody has to get on the same page here, and take part of the responsibility for the caregiving."*

—*Michael McCrea, Ph.D.*

ADDRESSING UNAWARENESS WITH PATIENTS

Lack of awareness of deficits may be the most troubling aspect of Alzheimer disease and other dementia syndromes from a caregiver's perspective. When patients are unaware of their deficits and feel physically fine, they do not perceive themselves as patients in need of care, or vulnerable persons in need of protection. Care and protection may therefore be experienced as controlling, patronizing, or even something more sinister. Lack of awareness commonly results in resistance to the process of assessment, and certainly to hearing a diagnosis of dementia. (Additional strategies to address unawareness can be found in Chapter 12: Acquired Brain Injury.)

o *"Your mind is playing a trick on you. You can't remember that you can't remember."*

—*Susan McPherson, Ph.D.*

o *"I know you think that there's not much wrong with you. But if I took 100 guys off the street, all as old as you are, went to school for the same amount of time, were all in the army as well ... you are doing worse than 99 of them. You are dead last. You had your own store. I am convinced that this is a change. This doesn't mean that we lock you up and throw away the key, but it does mean that we need to take this seriously."*

—*Jacobus Donders, Ph.D.*

Joining with patient's unawareness

Oftentimes, the patient's unawareness of deficit has to be addressed before the patient will even be willing to participate in the testing process. Their unshakable conviction that nothing is wrong may lead to a refusal to be evaluated. This pearl may be used prior to testing:

o *"It's a win/win situation. If you do well on the memory testing, like you think you will, then you get your daughter/wife off your back. If the testing shows some memory problems, we get you some help for them. Either way, it's a win/win situation."*

—*Karen Postal, Ph.D.*

Helping an unaware patient buy into compensatory strategies

o *(Said to patient and caregiver together)*—*"I know you are both disagreeing on how well your memory works. You get into arguments over it. I'm sure that doesn't make for a very pleasant home environment. So I'm going to make some suggestions that might eliminate some of the arguments you have.*

o *"I want you to start religiously using a calendar to write things down: doctor's appointments, lunch with Cousin Peter, a plan to see your grandkids next Thursday. Don't just tell each other about it, when you say 'this event is happening on Thursday,' go and write everything on the calendar, or show your spouse that it is written on the calendar. If you use a calendar, where you write things down, if your wife actually hasn't told you about the event, then you can prove it to her! It won't be on the calendar!*

o *"In the same way, I want you to start using a medicine organizer. If you use a medicine organizer, and she's telling you that you forgot to take the meds, you can prove to her you did."*

—John Lucas, Ph.D.

Addressing patient unawareness with caregivers

o *(To caregivers)*—*"One of the blessings of Alzheimer disease is lack of insight. But it's also a curse. The blessing is that they don't have to mourn their loss of memory and thinking abilities. But the curse is that they don't understand that they can't function as well and are not as safe."*

—Cynthia Kubu, Ph.D.

o *"Your husband may think that he is capable of things that he clearly is not. It's important not to try to convince him of his difficulties or say, 'I am going to do this because you can't.' That will set the stage for power struggles and arguments. It is often better to just offer assistance than to convince him he can't do something."*

—Joel Rosenbaum, Ph.D.

CAREGIVER UNAWARENESS AND DENIAL

At times, caregivers may also demonstrate a lack of awareness of their spouse's or family member's deficits. This can result in patients not receiving appropriate medical treatment and practical support in day-to-day life. In these instances, a primary purpose, if not *the* primary purpose, of the feedback session is to help the family understand the seriousness of their loved one's impairments.

The Texas Functional Living Scale includes real-world activities like writing checks. Sometimes in a dementia feedback, a patient's daughter might say, "Well, I couldn't memorize that list of words either," indicating that she didn't feel the patient was really that bad off. Oftentimes this is a family member who does not live close to the patient. Sharing a concrete task from the testing that the patient could not do is often helpful to break though family denial. Showing the results to the family can be very powerful.

- o *"Well, as part of the evaluation we asked your dad to write a check to the water company. To pay the bill and record it in the check ledger—he couldn't do it. See? Here's what he did ... he made the check out to 'Bill' when I asked him to pay the bill. He also could not address an envelope or make correct change from a one-dollar bill."*

  —Munro Cullum, Ph.D.

- o *Sometimes, the spouse is still interacting with the patient as if they did not have any functional memory difficulties. They are also getting very upset with them for not remembering, or for not using reason. I will sometimes pull out a three- or four-word memory task and administer it in front of the spouse. I even write the words down and let the patient hold the list. When they can't remember hearing the words but have them in their hand, the spouse gets it. "You see? He really can't remember these things. I even wrote the words down for him."*

  —Jim Irby, Ph.D.

Sometimes family members who do not live near the patient believe that the patient is adapting quite well based on the information they are able to glean through frequent (or intermittent) phone calls. I like to use this example to demonstrate how hard it is to get accurate information through a phone call—it often takes a number of questions to find out there is a problem.

- o *"Families often tell me, 'Well, we call and they're fine.' Well, I'll tell you a story about calling. My wife used to call my mother-in-law regularly, and at the end of the call she would say 'can I talk to Dad before we hang up?' Her mother would say, 'well, I can't put him on the phone, he's in the living room.'*

  'Well why can't you put him on the phone? Is he alright?'
  'Yeah, he's fine.'
  'Then bring the phone to the living room so we can talk.'
  'Well he's on the floor and he can't get up.'

  You have to ask that many questions to get the information, 'he's fine, he's in the living room, but he's on the floor.' You can't learn from the phone how they are doing."

  —Tom Boll, Ph.D.

There's always a family member who doesn't want to put a parent in a nursing home. But they're often not the one who takes care of her. They object to the primary caretaker's assessment of the patient's disability as well as their thoughts on intervention. The problem is, they are not there to witness the patient's cognitive limitations, nor are they the ones who are actually caring for the patient.

o *"Let's allow Mom to visit the relative who doesn't think she needs it. Let's put Mom on a plane: you may have to go with her, but Mom's going to visit for a week, and then let's have the conversation. If she's fine there, great! Let's see what they're doing! I'd love to be wrong here, but I'm not. These family members need to have the experience of your mother, and they're not."*

—Tom Boll, Ph.D.

DRIVING

There are situations in which a patient's lack of insight is harmful to themselves and their family. Driving is certainly one of those instances. Conversations about driving safety can be very difficult, and highly charged. Depending on the patient's stage of dementia, he or she can leave the office and immediately forget the conversation. This is not a reason to "skip" the topic, however. Indeed, talking to patients about driving is a perfect opportunity to model the conversation for family members, especially since the discussion will almost certainly have to take place repeatedly once the feedback session is over. Clinicians model how to be simultaneously firm, reasonable, and reassuring by employing an authoritative but sympathetic tone of voice.

Differentiating between operating a vehicle and safe driving

o *"I have no doubt that you know how to operate a motor vehicle. I have no doubt that you know what to do when you sit down in a car—to turn it on and drive. What I am concerned about is your memory. When you are driving, because of your memory, you are likely to forget where you are going. And when that happens, you lose attention to the road, and that raises your likelihood of having an accident. Your ability to drive in traffic in a safe fashion is compromised by your memory. So I need to make the recommendation that you can't drive."*

—John Lucas, Ph.D.

Left hand turn metaphor for safe driving

When the issue of driving arises, often patients and family members minimize the risk of driving by saying, "But he only drives to the grocery store and back." The following is an effective way of reminding families how inherently demanding driving is. This can be expanded as necessary to include very detailed descriptions of how patients must be visually alert to other cars while still paying appropriate attention to their own driving.

o *"Think about all that goes into making a left-hand turn across traffic. You're judging your own speed, and your own reaction time. At the same time, you are judging the other cars' speed. A lot goes into it."*

—Mark Barisa. Ph.D.

Safe driving: would you put your grandchild in the back seat?

Family members will often say that the patient has always been so independent that it would "kill him" if they took away the keys to the car. Sometimes family members are so concerned about taking things away from the patient that they are willing to diminish the driving safety issue.

o *"As long as you feel safe with your grandchild in the back seat of that car, I would say that it's your choice. But if you have any concern about having your grandchild in the back seat I would think twice about it. Because you are not only putting your own grandkids at risk when he is driving them, you are putting other peoples' grandchildren at risk as well."*

—John Lucas, Ph.D.

Safe driving: empowering spouses

When discussing driving you need to be direct. No pussyfooting. The real deal is talking to the spouse, because the burden is on him or her to make sure the patient doesn't drive.

o *"You have the problem of what to do with the keys. Sometimes you have to hide the keys and then live with that. There's that period in many dementias when the patient's behavior is extremely difficult to manage and the patient can no longer reason well or appreciate his/her deficits."*

—Muriel D, Lezak, Ph.D.

o *(To the caregivers)—"Some people genuinely don't recall the conversation in which they agreed not to drive, or they are wily, they just take the keys and go. Bottom line is you can't be there all the time to police them. You will need to hide the keys, or disconnect the battery or sparkplug wire."*

—John Lucas, Ph.D.

Because reasoning skills in an Alzheimer patient are impaired, they are likely to be unable to make appropriate decisions about driving, etc. They often react to the restriction in a childlike way, "She is preventing me from driving." It's helpful to put the message in black-and-white terms.

o *"This is not about some kind of a fight or dispute you have with your wife"* (or son). *"This is about safety. Your safety and the safety of others."*

—Aaron Nelson, Ph.D.

Framing driving test as a favor

o *"I'm really concerned about your driving. But I'll go to bat for you and get you a driving test. If you pass the test you can drive. I'm not concerned that you are going to drive recklessly, but I worry about the time when the kid runs after a ball in front of your car, and you won't be fast enough to stop. And you would never forgive yourself."*

—Jacobus Donders, Ph.D.

Emphasizing liability issues when discussing safe driving

o *"I'm going to put in my report that in my opinion, your impairments in visuo-perception are big enough that you are incurring a big risk when driving. If you continue to drive, you are putting yourself at risk for being sued. This is the United States. Everyone sues everyone else. Do you want to put your family at risk for that? Ninety percent of the time, you're just fine. But if something unexpected happens, and you get into an accident—and they find out that you were told not to drive, you could lose everything. You may not be fully aware of it, but the testing shows it's not safe for you to drive."*

—Christopher Randolph, Ph.D.

o *"Look, I'm going to be the bad guy here. I am going to put in my report that you aren't able to drive. And once I do you are liable in a suit if you do drive."*

—Christopher Randolph, Ph.D.

o *"Insurance policies have this little fine print—you know, none of us ever even get a copy, much less read our insurance policy. Your insurance agent's secretary (because he's out golfing!) just says you're covered. But all the policies say that you agree to not drive in an impaired condition. So if you have a physician that has given an indication that you are impaired, then the insurance company doesn't have to pay."* (Hit him in the pocket book). *"But if you go to a driving eval, and were told you could do this, now you have negated that issue."*

—Mark Barisa, Ph.D.

Safe driving: helping patients find a ride

o *"This is a liability issue. You have documented cognitive problems. If you get into an accident, you will lose everything. You'll lose the shirt off your back. This will affect your wife, your kids. So, if you can't drive any longer, how do we maintain that independence and mobility you have now?" "Okay, so Dad plays cards every Thursday. Let's have one of the guys pick him up. Who will drive him to church every Sunday?"*

—Michael McCrea, Ph.D.

Safe driving: using macabre photos to break through resistance

o *"One of my primary goals is to help you maintain your independence, but we need to balance that with your potential to hurt someone. Here, I want to show you this article"* (hands patient a newspaper article with very gory picture of pedestrian vs. car accident).

—*Michael Santa Maria, Ph.D.*

Legacy metaphor for safe driving

o *"I know in this country driving is our ticket to independence. But you don't want your legacy to be 'the guy who ran over the kid on the bicycle.' I remember about three years ago an older person lost control of their car at O'Hare. Drove right through the front of the airport, right into the building. And my first gut reaction was, he might have worked 50 years as a schoolteacher, he has 27 grandkids. But he's going to die as 'the guy who ran into O'Hare Airport.' You don't want to be the guy who ran over the kid on the bicycle."*

—*Michael McCrea, Ph.D.*

Safe driving: taking the blame for taking the keys

I'm looking to be the bad guy, trying to deflect conflict between the patient and family onto myself. It's not "you're trying to take my keys." Rather, it becomes, "Dr. Nelson took the keys from you," or "Dr. Nelson said you can't be alone, or manage your medication." Because their reasoning is poor, they are likely to experience this limitation as a power struggle within the family. As clinicians, we can be the bad guys, because we are not the people who have to then provide the care for the next 10 years. Caregivers can just point to us. Put our pictures on the wall and throw darts at it, I don't care. If it helps the family in their role as care providers for the patient, then I've done my job.

o *"Look, this is not your family saying this. This is me. If you want to be angry at someone for this, be angry at me. This is the way it's going to have to be. From now on, your daughter is going to give you your medicines twice a day. From now on you're not going to be driving a car. The car will be gone. It's really horrible— blame me. I just want you to know I'm not doing this out of spite."*

—*Aaron Nelson, Ph.D.*

SECURING SERVICES IN THE HOME AND TRANSITIONING TO ASSISTED LIVING OR NURSING HOME PLACEMENT

Closely related to lack of awareness is a patient's tendency to reject help in their daily lives. Mothers fire housekeepers their children have hired. Patients feel insulted when their spouse tries to organize their medications. Although they might be unable to take care of their own basic needs, patients, and at times family members, often will also reject the notion that they need an assisted living facility.

Helping patients accept help

o *"Let's not argue about the extent of the deficits. Let's talk about some reasonable precautions. I don't think you need a babysitter, but how about someone looking in on you a couple of times a day. Can it be by phone?"*

—*Jacobus Donders, Ph.D.*

Many patients are so impaired that they could not have this type of conversation. But occasionally I get a college-educated person who is interested and insightful. My emphasis in these circumstances is proactive management.

o *"When you came in, you were insisting that your memory was just fine. The testing showed there was a problem. And that's normal, because when you have a problem with memory your brain doesn't let you know about it. But other people see it. So I want you to rely more on your niece to help you with some things that involve memory—to make sure you don't have a problem. People who score the way you did on these memory tests frequently have problems paying bills, like paying twice, or problems with taking medicine. These are the things that you need someone to help you with oversight. So to begin with, let's put you on automatic payment with your bills."*

—*Christopher Randolph, Ph.D.*

There are some differences in providing feedback to male versus female patients. Oftentimes, the male has spent his whole life being the patriarch of the family—in control. Taking the car keys away, or having someone else handle the finances can feel diminishing. The construct "now it's time to sit back and be waited on" turns the situation into a traditional honor instead of a submissive role.

o *"You've given your entire life to the family. It's time to reap the benefits. It's time to sit in that recliner and let them wait on you."*

—*Mark Barisa, Ph.D.*

When dementia patients refuse help, it is time to start the bargaining process. Bring in motivational interviewing. "Here's the problem: what are you going to do about it?" Recruit the patient as part of the solution.

o *"Do you think one of those Lifeline buttons would be good for you?"*

—*Mark Barisa, Ph.D.*

o *"I know you are good with your medicines 95 percent of the time. But I worry that with some of these meds you need to be right 100 percent of the time. Heck, I forget meds myself sometimes. My wife has to remind me. Do yourself a favor and let your wife remind you."*

—*Jacobus Donders, Ph.D.*

o *"Accepting help is difficult for many patients, particularly if they have been in the role of the caregiver all of their lives. If people are willing to help you, that's a blessing to them. Think of how good you feel when you are able to give to someone. By accepting help, you are giving your family a gift."*

—*Cynthia Kubu, Ph.D.*

Helping caregivers create a caregiver plan

o *"I've already provided feedback to your dad" (walk family members through the diagnosis). "This is not a crisis. Your dad will leave here in no worse shape than yesterday, based on this diagnosis. For some families, I say, your dad can't go home and live by himself tonight. But that's not the case here. Your father can go home and live on his own. But over time, he will need more assistance to maintain himself at home. The goal here is to keep you ahead of the curve so you don't have a crisis. Don't wait until a crisis occurs to talk together about how more supports will be added so your father can function well."*

—*Michael McCrea, Ph.D.*

Placing a loved one in a nursing home

The decision about nursing home placement is really hard. Often family members will say, "But we told him we would never send him to a nursing home!" A helpful construct to inject into those conversations is: "Safety is more important than promises."

o *"We make a lot of promises to family members. Ninety-nine percent of them we can keep. Think about when you were a parent. Sometimes you had to break a promise to one of your kids. This is about his safety. You made a promise to him, sure. But if he had made a promise to you, and he knew that breaking that promise to you would put you in danger ... he would break that promise."*

—*Michael McCrea, Ph.D.*

o *"I know how hard this is. I have to have discussions like this frequently. And I'll be the guy that, the day they try to move me out of my house, I'll be sitting there with a shotgun. Over my dead body!"*

—*Michael McCrea, Ph.D.*

o *"Go see these places. You have a vision of what nursing homes were like 30 years ago. They're not the same. I remember visiting nursing homes with my mom and dad 30 years ago—and holy Toledo! They're not like that."*

—Michael McCrea, Ph.D.

HELPING PATIENTS AND CAREGIVERS ACCEPT AND IMPLEMENT COMPENSATORY STRATEGIES

When trying to convince caregivers to get patients into the habit of using calendars and compensatory strategies, they may argue that it is easier just to tell them what day it is. In these cases I emphasize:

o *"You are trying to get them into the habit. When you develop the habits and routines they stick. The earlier you get into the habit in the disease process the better."*

—John Lucas, Ph.D.

o *"If you had a problem with memory and you had to look at this calendar and figure out when you are going out to dinner with the Smiths—if you don't know what day it is, and seeing all this info, it's really hard to figure out."* (Then show them a calendar with days X'd out). *"See how much easier this is to figure out what we are doing today? You will be responsible to put an X on the previous day. Now when they go to the calendar, they will easily see what day they are on, what is the day's plan, and it will even anchor them to what happened yesterday."*

—John Lucas, Ph.D.

Presidential assistant metaphor to help patients accept compensatory strategies

Patients with memory problems can self-isolate to avoid potentially embarrassing situations. Many patients also see compensatory strategies as things that mark them as stupid or needy. This analogy shifts this negative perspective by focusing on how very-high-status individuals need to use compensation strategies as well.

o *"You know, President Obama"* (or Bush, with a Republican patient) *"walks into a room, and he doesn't know anyone's name either. He's looking at a ballroom full of 100 diplomats and senators and he doesn't want to insult anyone by not remembering their name. He has a presidential aide who stands by his side and whispers, 'Mr. President, that's Admiral Smith, he met you three years ago at....' Well, that must be how it feels sometimes when you go to the senior center—a room full of people you can't remember. You can enlist your best friend"* (or husband) *"to be your presidential advisor. They can just stick close and whisper, 'Oh, that's Jane Smith, she plays bridge with…. '"*

—Karen Postal, Ph.D.

Paying attention to the patient's emotion—strategies for the caregiver

○ *"What I am asking you to do is very unnatural. It's very easy for me to sit here and describe, and I recognize that this is a very hard thing to do. For someone with dementia, sometimes you don't want to pay attention to the words coming out of their mouth, but to their emotions. I am going to ask you to agree first, to whatever they say. No matter how crazy it sounds. Say, 'I can see what you mean when you explain it like that.' Or 'You're right, I can see why you would think that.' When your wife is saying something that is completely untrue, or totally crazy, like 'Uncle Joe stole my purse,' try and stay real calm and say, 'You're right, he may have stolen your purse. I can see why that would be upsetting, let's try to find it.' Then you get into redirecting. 'Yeah, we need to look for that, but why don't we do this first.' Or, 'Yes, I think she may have taken your purse but I really need your help first, Can you help me fold this laundry?' Or, 'Okay, lets go look for it,' (and while in the other room, change the subject). Try and have some kind of standard or simple task ready that you know they don't mind doing. When someone is agitated, quit trying to reason. Stay calm, and pay more attention to how they are feeling. It's not a natural way to respond and it's really hard to do when you need to be somewhere or get something done. But choose your battles, and with practice you can get better at focusing more on how they're feeling instead of what they're saying."*

—Jim Irby, Ph.D.

Reminding patients that quality of life does not require a good memory

○ *"You don't need a good memory to have a good quality of life. You can live a very fulfilling day-to-day life with absolutely no memory as long as you're prepared for it—as long as you can compensate for it. There are a number of things we can do in your day-to-day activities that will minimize problems associated with not being able to remember well"* (at this point, data collected from interview can be brought in, e.g., help with meds, online banking, calls to remember). *"Have you considered…. "*

—John Lucas, Ph.D.

○ *"Your social graces are wonderful. It was a delight to interact with you. I bet everyone who interacts with you really enjoys it. It's important to have as many social interactions as possible, because that's something you do well and enjoy. But we want to make sure that the interactions aren't turning into a memory test, or stressing your memory system too much."* (To caregiver)—*"It's helpful to give friends*

*and family a heads-up not to ask your wife to remember. Stay in the moment:
'That's a wonderful dress. You always look good in green …' (rather than asking,
'so, what did you do yesterday?')"*

—*John Lucas, Ph.D.*

MODELING NON-REACTIVE RESPONSES

We have all had the experience in a feedback session, of having an intense, earnest 30-minute conversation about the patient's visual and executive deficits and the need to take a driving evaluation before going back on the road, only to have the patient say, "Okay, Doc, this is all great. But I have a question. Can I drive?" Clearly, the patient has rapidly forgotten the entire conversation. Although of course this is frustrating, it is important to keep in mind that the conversation was beneficial to the caregivers who heard and will be able to act on the information. The moment also presents an excellent opportunity to model non-reactive responses to repeated questions. The key is to distill the basic message into a clear, authoritative sound bite that the caregivers can utilize as well.

o *"No, Mr. Smith. Because of changes in your brain you need to get a driving test before getting on the road, or your insurance won't cover you after an accident."*

—*Karen Postal, Ph.D.*

VISUAL HALLUCINATIONS AND CAPGRAS SYNDROMES

When clinicians ask about whether a patient has had visual hallucinations, often patients and family members are surprised. Patients may have been too embarrassed to tell anyone about the hallucinations, or feel that the hallucinations are a sign of insanity. The presence of hallucinations or delusional misidentification symptoms can create distance and alienation between patients and their families, who may begin treating the patients as "crazy." Simple explanations of how brain changes associated with dementia or other processes may cause hallucinations can be very reassuring; patients and families typically feel relieved to attribute the symptoms to structural brain damage.

o *"People with Parkinson's have hallucinations. I can tell you that many people that I directly ask about them don't tell me. But they have them. It's a well-known effect of the disease. And of course they aren't real. It's your brain playing tricks on you and it's because you have Parkinson's. It's an effect of the disease."*

—*Roberta F. White, Ph.D.*

o *"Your mother has a symptom with a very fancy name: reduplicative paramnesia. It means she thinks there is an exact copy of her house somewhere else, and sometimes she feels that she is in that remote location. It sounds crazy, but your mother is not crazy. This is a symptom that, believe it or not, is pretty common in the context of the changes in the brain brought on by"* (fill in the blank: Alzheimer disease, stroke …).

"The visual processing system has to work really hard every time we enter a room to figure out what we are seeing—it's a huge amount of data. It's done unconsciously—we never know we do it. And it happens really rapidly. Your mother's visual processing system will occasionally make mistakes, and won't process some data (for example, furniture or wall placement) as feeling familiar. So she might have the sensation that she is in a copy of her house.

"Luckily, most of the time, just by taking a walk, and then returning, her visual processing system can get another chance to experience the house as familiar. Sometimes this technique works. Other times it doesn't."

—Karen Postal, Ph.D.

o *"How are you coping with this? How do you handle it when he is seeing something you don't? Do you try to talk him out of it? Sometimes if you go along with it, and think about what might make you feel better in that situation if it were real, that can help. So, if your wife is worried about an intruder, instead of trying to convince her that nobody is there, maybe it would be more reassuring to show her that you are checking the locks and doors? Try not to argue. Instead try to comment on the situation. For example, instead of pointing out that nobody is here, say, 'No, those kids won't be joining us.' If the patient does not know you, leave the room and then return, announcing your return, or just go along with it: 'Yup, I'm the good Louise. That other Louise had to leave.'"*

—Tanis Ferman, Ph.D.

o *"Sometimes it helps to ask, 'who does this behavior really bother?' Sometimes a hallucination is more upsetting to a family member, but does not really bother the person experiencing it. Ask yourself, is he scared by the images, is he behaving in an unsafe way, or are they really just a nuisance? If the behavior is really just a nuisance or annoyance, it may help to make a comment that is more inquiring or reassuring: 'Is that dog back again? He must like you.'"*

—Tanis Ferman, Ph.D.

When a patient is experiencing hallucinations but is too demented or unable to understand a brain-based explanation, it's better to have a pleasant experience, rather than creating a moment of anxiety through confrontation. Although I might have a separate discussion with the family or conservators.

o *"Oh! Who's there?" ("My ex-husband.") "How's he doing!?"*

—Robert M. Bilder, Ph.D.

Dementia severity and hallucinations

With Capgras syndrome, patients believe family members look the same on the outside but have been replaced on the inside by someone else (i.e., an imposter). Families may understandably misinterpret the presence of Capgras syndrome or other delusional misidentification symptoms as reflecting an advanced dementia stage. It can be very reassuring to clarify that this isn't the case.

> o *"This symptom doesn't seem very well tied to the severity of the dementia. These things can kind of crop up on their own, and they're relatively common. About half of those with Alzheimer disease will have delusions in the course of the disease."*
> —*Mark Bondi, Ph.D.*

LEGAL ISSUES

Explaining capacity evaluations

> o *There's the formation of a Power of Attorney (POA) and then there's the activation. My way of understanding whether a health care Power of Attorney should be activated is as simple as, "If he were to come to this hospital alone tomorrow afternoon. No family members were around—he had to be brought here by ambulance—and in the ER they determined that he needed a procedure done, could he understand the information and make a decision about whether or not having the procedure was in his best interest? And if I start to have a concern about whether he is able to do that—then it's time to give proper authorization to the health care POA to do that.*
> —*Michael McCrea, Ph.D.*

7 Attention Deficit Hyperactivity Disorder

BECAUSE ITS CORE deficit includes executive dysfunction, explaining the impact of attention deficit hyperactivity disorder (ADHD) on a patient's daily functioning incorporates multiple aspects of a neuropsychologist's knowledge base. For this reason, many of the pearls explaining inattention and poor executive function in this chapter are equally appropriate for utilization in other populations, such as those suffering from traumatic brain injury (TBI).

ADHD's high incidence rate and frequent appearance as a topic in the popular media also means that patients and families may walk in with misconceptions and beliefs that can make diagnosis and treatment recommendations difficult to accept. This chapter offers effective strategies to assist clinicians in clarifying core deficits and engaging patients and family members in "owning" diagnoses and treatment plans. Although most of the pearls were presented from the context of a pediatric practice, they generally translate well for feedback session with adults who have been diagnosed with ADHD.

DEFINING ATTENTION PROBLEMS

What constitutes an "attention problem?" Helping patients and families understand the concept of developmentally appropriate attention skills is a challenge, especially when these problems are accompanied by the tendency to hyperfocus on preferred activities, such as videogames, television, Legos, or even reading. When individuals hyperfocus, others may assume that this is evidence that ADHD could not be a possibility.

Explaining difficulties with sustained mental effort

I use this metaphor to explain how ADHD interferes with a child's ability to just sit down and work. It's a good way to explain difficulties with sustained mental effort, as well as attention difficulties—although it isn't always as effective when one of the parents is an accountant.

o *"Most children don't like doing homework—they do it, but it's not like they are running home all excited to spend more time with their books. But, for most kids, doing homework is a lot like balancing your checkbook. If you're anything like me, this is something you have to do, but it's not all that onerous. You sit down, do it, and get it over with.*

"For kids who have ADHD, doing homework is a lot more like doing your taxes" (and depending on how heavy I feel I have to be to make the point, I may add ... "after you've been up all night and I won't let you have any coffee"). *"Suddenly, you are looking to do all those things that you normally avoid, like doing the laundry, mowing the lawn, cleaning the bathroom—anything but doing those taxes! That's what it's like every day your child sits down to do his homework—it takes him a great deal of effort just to sit himself down at the table and stay there, let alone do his work."*

—*Kira Armstrong, Ph.D.*

Blood pressure metaphor for attention

o *"Yes, these are all symptoms we all exhibit to some degree, just like blood pressure. We all have blood pressure—sometimes it's a little too high, so maybe we're advised to watch it, to exercise more, to adjust our daily routines and schedules to accommodate it, just like we might suggest to someone with just a little trouble focusing, or with impulse control. But, like everything else on a continuum"* (draw a line), *"there comes that magical point where we pronounce it as 'high,' and we give it a name and sometimes treat it with a pill.*

We have the same continuum for ADHD. And, like high blood pressure, ADHD can vary over time, in terms of its severity, or even whether it has a significant impact on our lives, depending on other things we do to accommodate, or treat it."

—Marla Shapiro, Ph.D.

Shiny object metaphor for distractibility

o *"Attention deficit disorder is a really misleading name for what's going on in the brain of kids and adults with ADHD. Our primitive attention system is literally hardwired to pay attention to things that are new and shiny. Babies automatically focus attention on things that are new and bright"* (demonstrate by holding fingers in front of my eyes from one angle, then the next). *"You dangle something new in front of a baby, and she will look at it. Then you dangle something newer, and she will look at that thing."*

(Use a 3-D brain model to demonstrate): *"This part of the brain is called the frontal lobe. It's the last part of the brain to develop, and its job is to override the primitive attention system. The frontal lobe helps kids pay attention to the thing they need to do to reach a goal, rather than the most interesting thing in the room. As children's frontal systems grow, they develop the ability to drag their attention away from the newest, shiniest, most interesting thing in the room to things that are less intrinsically interesting, but are important to meet goals. Such as seatwork, or studying. And each year kids can do this better. Third-graders are better than kindergarteners at seatwork, and high school kids can focus for much longer periods of time than fifth-graders.*

"With ADD, it's not that Rebecca's frontal lobe isn't working at all, she's much better at dragging her attention away from her favorite pastimes (like Legos) than she used to be when there is work to be done. It's just that she's not able to do this as well as the typical kid her age. And that's the disability. Many people feel it should really be called the 'directing-your-attention disorder.'"

—Karen Postal, Ph.D.

Hyperfocusing

o *"It's not that your child can't pay attention at all. Indeed, one thing that comes with ADHD is the tendency to hyperfocus. For example, some children with ADHD can play video games until their hands fall off, watch TV until their eyes pop out, or if they like to read, they may spend all night under their covers with a flashlight. The problem with ADHD is that they struggle to sustain their attention when they are being asked to do something outside of their preferred area of interest."*

—*Kira Armstrong, Ph.D.*

Barkley's concept of directed attention is helpful in explaining why hyperfocusing can be present in people who have ADHD.

o *"It's not that you can't pay attention, it's that it's disproportionally difficult for you to pay attention to something that doesn't grab your attention."*

—*Robb Mapou, Ph.D.*

Attention is not a passive process

This helps families understand why movement can actually facilitate the learning process in ADHD.

o *"It's really telling—when you ask a child with ADHD to lie still in a brain scanner. All they are asked to do is 'lie still, don't think about anything. Close your eyes and relax.' And you give that instruction to other children without ADHD too. The kids with ADHD are activating a lot of their cortex—especially their frontal cortex. The kids without ADHD are not.*

"So sitting still is an active cognitive process for these kids. They have to work hard to sit still and work hard to overcome their desire to move. If sitting still is an active cognitive process, and we have a limited amount of cognitive processing we can use at any one time—and if you are a teacher, asking them to sit still and learn a task, you are using up cognitive resources that otherwise could be used to learn the task." (This explanation really helps teachers.) "If you believe that, then how do the 'sit up straight and pay attention' demands of class interfere with learning? And how can we use movement, which is a more natural process for these kids, to help their cognitive efficiency?"

—*E. Mark Mahone, Ph.D.*

Gifted and ADHD

When providing feedback, it is important to pitch the level and content of the message to the parents' culture, socioeconomic status, and education level. Providing feedback to highly educated parents, such as university professors, can be challenging. I recall working with two professors of Chinese descent who had adopted a boy from China. They felt he was "just" bright and bored. In fact, it was my clinical opinion that he really had ADHD. They were both resistant to the idea, although the fact that they had brought him in suggested to me that they were genuinely concerned that they might be wrong. I had to take them through the feedback process with small steps.

o *"Help me with this disconnect.... Your son is really bright and he wants to please you. Would you agree he wants to please you? Then why would he be getting in trouble at school? Typically bright kids figure out another way, if they are bored in class, rather than getting in trouble."*

—Robin Hilsabeck, Ph.D.

o *"Imagine that you are preparing an elegant dinner for 20—say, Thanksgiving dinner. You must plan the menu, make a shopping list, invite the guests, and prepare the food so it all comes out on time. These are executive functions—planning, problem solving, time estimation, time management—that are part of the weakness for people with ADHD. Now—imagine that you have purchased the finest ingredients money can buy for your dinner. However, if the chef falls asleep (like in the movie Julie and Julia) or doesn't plan well, the meal will be ruined. A gifted person with ADHD has excellent ingredients, but the chef isn't always available." (Sometimes I say "the chef went out to lunch.")*

—Judith Glasser, PhD

EXPLAINING THE DIFFERENCE BETWEEN CAN'T AND WON'T

Children with ADHD often engage in impulsive, distracted, dysregulated behaviors that can disrupt the day-to-day lives of their entire family. Often these children engage in the same repetitive behaviors even when told to stop—leading parents to believe they are doing them intentionally or that they don't care what others think or feel about them. Helping parents differentiate between oppositional behaviors (which may also be present) and the consequences of ADHD can help them build different mental sets, which in turn helps them better tolerate their child's symptoms.

Mistake making machine metaphor for impulsivity

This helps dissuade families from the idea that their child can be educated into being better. It helps them recognize that this is a *performance* deficit, not a knowledge deficit.

o *"Children with ADHD elicit enormous amounts of correction from the adults in their environment, but this is a performance deficit, it isn't a skill deficit. David knows what he should do. The problem is he's not capable of doing it in the moment when it's time to do it. People with ADHD all have organizers. Probably more than one PDA" (personal digital assistant). "And they all know how to use them. The problem is not about the skill of using the PDA. It's the performance of using it in the moment when they should be putting the appointment into it. Poor David—we see the teacher's report. He is really having the experience of being a mistake-making machine. What's life like for him? He's just out there 'David-ing around,' and he keeps getting into trouble because he's doing stuff and he's not even realizing what he's done. He wouldn't do it if he had full awareness and full executive control—he wouldn't do the things he does that elicit all this correction. But he can't help it, so of course he feels like a mistake-making machine."*

—*Steve Hughes, Ph.D.*

Driving uphill metaphor for ADHD

This metaphor helps explain why individuals with ADHD can *sometimes* do things and then sometimes cannot, or why more complex tasks are so challenging.

o *"It's like gas in the gas tank … do you use more gas in the same car at the same speed traveling uphill or downhill? Of course, you use more gas going uphill, because it's more effortful. Think about how hard it is for Susie to get through her day, how much gas she has to use just to stay focused—it's like her car's going uphill all day, and she just runs out of gas. She just can't keep expending that level of energy, day in and day out, with no breaks and no help. So, anything we can use to make getting through the day less effortful, like sitting her up front so that focusing isn't as hard, or giving her a routine so that remembering to write down assignments isn't as hard, will help her get through the day using less gas, so that she has more energy left for the things that really matter, and can use that 'gas' where it's most needed. Letting her play at recess instead of finishing up her seatwork, that's like refilling her tank—giving her a break to literally refuel."*

—*Marla Shapiro, Ph.D.*

Learned helplessness

o *They have developed a learned helplessness. Part of the problem is that they don't know how to try. If they don't see the path, they can't take the first step.*

—*Steven Guy, Ph.D.*

Performance roller coaster metaphor for adhd

o *"For kids with ADHD, it's often like 'Whack-a–Mole,' constantly putting out fires. These kids are constantly dealing with problems—they are exhausted. When they are trying, they ride this roller coaster of performance. They start off the semester saying, 'I will do better this year.' And work really hard—but they have to put in much more time in than the typical kid. They run out of gas—they get exhausted. Then the teachers and parents are upset: 'But they could do it last week—why are they so inconsistent?' It's a roller coaster of performance for them. They might start giving up."*

o (*Turns to kid*): *"We can smooth this out for you and make things more consistent. If you do this tutoring and executive function stuff, you will get 1000 percent return on this."*

—Steven Guy, Ph.D.

EXECUTIVE FUNCTIONS

"Executive function" can be a difficult concept for family members to understand. This confusion often leads to incorrect attributions about the patient's behavior and intentions. For example, parents can become confused about seemingly new academic and social problems when their children have historically been able to compensate for their difficulties. Adults may experience anger from spouses or co-workers who are frustrated with their lack of follow-through, inconsistent performance, and seeming lack of desire to change these problems. These pearls below provide metaphors to help explain the role of executive functions, and what happens when they are impaired. We have included several that have overlapping themes, with the idea that you will be able to select and/or modify the one that best suits your own practice. (Additional pearls for executive functions can also be found in Chapter 5: "Putting Feedback to Work with Patients from Multiple Populations.")

Bosses and workers metaphor for executive functions

o *"The brain is composed of two parts: You've got the workers and you've got the bosses. In ADHD, what happens is that you have a lot of workers. But those workers are an unruly bunch. If the bosses aren't on top of them, the workers do all kinds of bad stuff. In ADHD, the bosses are asleep. They are in the office goofing off, not paying attention to the workers. The workers are doing all kinds of inappropriate things and not being very productive, they need to have the boss do his or her job—manage the workers."*

—James Brad Hale, Ph.D.

The brain-boss metaphor can be extended to explain inconsistencies in a person's day-to-day behaviors.

o *"What's consistent about ADHD is that there are lots of inconsistencies. The variability depends on whether the bosses are doing their jobs that day or not. Jack might be doing something well Monday. His brain bosses are on the job. But on Tuesday, he doesn't do the thing well. His bosses are off duty."*

—James Brad Hale, Ph.D.

The brain-boss metaphor can also be extended to explain oppositional behaviors.

o *"John misbehaves a lot. He does a lot of the wrong things. I'm not trying to say that this brain boss thing is an excuse. A 'no' is still a 'no.' But what the medication will do is allow his brain bosses time to stop and think. 'If I do x, y, z, what will happen?' John still needs to be parented. And he still needs consequences for his actions.*

But what happens when he's not on medication and he does something wrong? If you ask him, 'Was [that] the right thing to do?' Most ADHD kids can tell you, 'No, it wasn't.' They understand what they are supposed to do. But, if you ask him why he did it, he will say, 'I don't know.' A lot of teachers and parents feel the kid is being noncompliant at that point. But you have to keep in mind, when he said, 'I don't know,' he may really not know. He didn't think to do the right thing because the brain boss didn't say at that moment, 'Hey, don't do that!'

"Let me give you an example of this kid, who during transition times (e.g., recess, lunchtime) would shove other kids in line. So we developed an intervention: when you are in line, put your hands in your pockets. And it worked very well. Then one day, he didn't and he shoved another kid, and got into a big fight. The teacher came over, and yelled, 'Joey! What were you supposed to do!?' Joey sheepishly replied, 'I was supposed to put my hands in my pockets.' And a little tear came out of his eye. It's not that he doesn't know. The boss was off duty and it wasn't a volitional action."

—*James Brad Hale, Ph.D.*

Executive secretary metaphor for executive functions

o *"The executive function system is like an executive secretary for the brain, who is the CEO. The secretary's job is to screen information coming into the CEO—like sorting mail, and sifting through emails, and packages that come in. She's [he's] also responsible for prioritizing. What goes on the brain's desk? How it will be organized on the desk—in little chunks, in a file folder? Is it in the Tuesday folder where it should be, or did it get shoved into the Monday folder? Or is everything just all piled on the desk? So the brain can be really smart, but the secretary can be on too many coffee breaks, or out to lunch or really disorganized, and it will make the CEO look bad and function poorly."*

—*Jennifer Turek Queally, Ph.D.*

The executive secretary metaphor can be expanded to explain memory.

o *"The secretary is responsible for filing, and depending on how she has labeled the folder, that makes a difference in how information goes into memory and how easy it is to locate later. This is a good way to understand why a child can remember everything about Disney World, but seems to remember nothing from school. Three weeks prior to the Disney trip, you're talking about Disney every day—you've labeled the folder! 'Disney!!' And then you fly to a place that's called 'Disney.' Then you walk through the gate labeled 'Disney!' So you have labeled the folder, and it sparkles—the child can remember. In contrast, when you learn about World War II, you tend to mention the information one time, it tends to be a lot of information at once, and sometimes you might even make other folders labeled 'Hitler,' 'Europe,' etc. And maybe later that year, you read Anne Frank's diary and you may not even realize that should have gone into the World War II file. Maybe you never connect that until you visit the Holocaust museum at the age of 20—'I should have put those three together in one folder!' When kids are little, we are doing the integration and labeling for them. 'Oh, honey, that's a kitty!' (label) 'and that's a doggy! See, they're different. A kitty has ... and a doggy has ...' But around fourth grade we just stop labeling and integrating, and expect their brain to take over."*

—*Jennifer Turek Queally, Ph.D.*

The executive secretary metaphor can also be extended to address information overload. It can be meaningful for parents to walk out of a feedback session saying to themselves, "okay, my kid's executive secretary is on a coffee break right now, I just need to help him sort through the information...."

o *"So the executive secretary's other job is to not get completely overwhelmed when stuff comes in too fast—and give up and go for coffee. This seems to happen more often with slower processors. Too much information starts coming in and piling on the desk. The secretary gets overwhelmed and can't keep up—so she just gets up and goes to get coffee. When she comes back, there's too much to sort and organize. So, she takes some off the top, shoves it in a drawer, and then tries to start from there, or worse, just pushes it off the desk into the trash and keeps going. A lot of information gets lost in the process."*

—*Jennifer Turek Queally, Ph.D.*

Finally, the executive secretary metaphor can be extended to explain the impact of emotional distress.

o *"If the secretary is emotionally overwhelmed—for example, if she is stressed because her boyfriend broke up with her—she can't screen calls, she can't organize, etc. It is really challenging to multitask all day because of the focus on emotional feelings. So everything falls apart. If she's having a good day—she can tackle all the things she has been trained to do."*

—*Jennifer Turek Queally, Ph.D.*

Demystifying executive function

o *"We often refer to the types of difficulties you have with attention, organization, getting things done, getting started, knowing what to tune into or what not to tune into, as 'executive functions.' You might ask, what does that mean? Well, what does an executive do in a business? An executive has a lot of talent around him or her and has to decide what talent needs to be brought in, and when, to get the job done. The executive has to know what to tune into and what not to tune into; what's better left for later and what needs to be organized to get the task done. In some ways your brain is the same way. We've just done a lot of testing. We know you have a lot of strengths and talents, but the system involved in recruiting those strengths to get the job done is where you are having the difficulty."*

—*Joel Rosenbaum, Ph.D.*

○ *"Executive function is an unusual term. It is related to execution and getting the job done. It's so much more than sitting still and paying attention. The environment can shift. Bright kids' intellect can mask ADHD, but when the environment shifts, sometimes it can be obvious. Sarah did really well through third grade, but now that the environment at school has changed, and she is being asked to complete and organize a lot more work on her own, she isn't able to get the job done."*

—*Steven Guy, Ph.D.*

Car clutch metaphor for executive functions

○ *"Executive functions are those cognitive skills that help kids apply their reasoning skills in a particular task. They are like the clutch in your car. It doesn't matter how big or fancy an engine the car has, if the clutch doesn't work, the car won't go. So, it's kind of like that with executive functions and intelligence. You can be very intelligent, but if you have difficulty holding information or directions in mind long enough to follow them, the work won't get done. Executive function skills allow the work to get done and allow kids to demonstrate how 'smart' they really are."*

—*Lisa Jacobson, Ph.D.*

Sluggish cognitive tempo

○ *"The teacher will be saying 'a, b, c, d, e.' And your son will be thinking 'A … A … A … B … B … B … Oh my god! D! D … D … D …' Kids with ADHD are losing a lot of information by the nature of the fact that they are taking more time to process it."*

—*Bill MacAllister, Ph.D.*

TREATMENT ISSUES

Often parents struggle with the idea of putting their children on medication for ADHD. Some parents and patients have unrealistic hopes and expectations about the potential positive effects of medications. Other parents may be so focused on the potential side effects of stimulant medication that they completely ignore the possible benefits. This is most likely to occur if they have heard horror stories about children becoming "zombies," losing their creativity, or changing their personalities. Some parents view medication as a way of "drugging" children—something they are adamantly opposed to, no matter how much their children may be struggling with their ADHD symptoms. A subset of these parents, however, is more than willing to rely on "herbal ADHD medications" or other unregulated, unproven, and even potentially unsafe techniques. Cautioning families about these techniques without being dismissed as being part of the "corporate medical machine" can take finesse. Indeed, providing families with a balanced understanding of the potential benefits and side-effects of stimulants, as well as a clearer understanding of *why* medication might help, can be one of the most challenging, but important, tasks when working with this population.

Addressing stimulant "horror stories"

The overmedicated child who resembles a zombie is frequently brought up in consulting sessions with neuropsychologists who work with children with ADHD. "I don't want my child on drugs!" is a common refrain from parents. None of us want our children on drugs, but in those instances where it is clinically indicated, this message can help parents to become more open to the idea.

o *"Everybody loves to tell the 'horror' stories about Ritalin, but you rarely hear about the overwhelming majority of times it works. It's kind of like childbirth—no one talks about how they gave birth to their child in two hours and it was such a breeze, because let's face it ... we'd only hate them ... but the horror stories about long, painful childbirths—those get told all the time! We only hear the stimulant horror stories, because they are more 'fun' to tell."*
—*Kira Armstrong, Ph.D.*

Talking to parents about stimulants

o *"The medicine sets the table for the other things we need to do. It's a small piece of what we will do for your child. It doesn't organize his book bag, or organize his assignments. It allows him to be more available when we teach him to do these things. It's important for us to teach him to think about his thinking—because these kids tend not to do this. It's not like some teachers say—'Oh just put them on meds.' The intervention and treatment plan for ADHD is so much more."*
—*Steven Guy, Ph.D.*

o *"There are three types of parents: The first type say, 'For the love of God, please put my child on drugs so I don't have to parent them!' That's not a good place to be. The second type of parents say, 'There's no way I am going to put my kids on drugs.' And that's also not a good place to be. You seem to be in the center. No one likes to drug kids—put them on medications. But parents need to decide, and consider, 'here are the potential benefits, and drawbacks.'"*
—*Bill MacAllister, Ph.D.*

o *"I am a Ph.D., not an MD. You should talk to your physician about this. But it's worth considering, because it will set the table for John to be able to do what we know he can do. It can make a big difference. I've seen it make such a difference— I've had adolescents come back here and say thank you. I've just seen kids do better and feel more successful. I've seen kids have the slings and arrows reduced. They can have a different perspective on themselves and change their academic self-esteem."*
—*Steven Guy, Ph.D.*

o *"Look, what I usually hear is, 'Yeah we tried it, we felt it worked a little, then we upped the dose, and it worked a little.' But every once in a while, I hear, 'That was a magic bullet.' And maybe your child will be that child."*

—Bill MacAllister, Ph.D.

o *I tell parents, "I say this to every family that comes into my office—no matter why they are here. The most important thing for all kids is that they grow up feeling good about themselves. For me, I feel that it's time to consider medication if the ADHD is making them feel bad about themselves—socially, academically, or in their day-to-day interactions with you at home. If they are starting to think of themselves as stupid or 'bad,' or if their ADHD is interfering in their ability to make or keep friends, then it's time to consider medication."*

—Kira Armstrong, Ph.D.

o *"I'm pretty conservative with medication. Not every child that walks through the door needs to be on medication. You came to see me because you wanted a broader assessment than what might be done by your pediatrician. Your child was with us for six hours, and we looked at attention in lots of different ways. We were able to get a very good picture of what is happening with his attention and learning.*

I start to think about medication when attention is interfering with your child's learning. This is the picture I am hearing from you and the teacher—and what we saw in here during testing." (Or, "I'm not hearing you say that—but if you start to hear that, that's when you might want to start thinking about medication.")

—Jennifer Janusz, Psy.D.

o *"Let's say the average child can sit in class and pay attention for 45 minutes. If Johnny can only pay attention for a portion of that, the rest is essentially time lost. It's like he's essentially not in school for that time."*

—Bill MacAllister, Ph.D.

Early in my career I would be willing to engage in what, in retrospect, I would call an argument about medication. But as I matured, I no longer engage in arguments about that. I am interested in seeing the child and the parents again, and they may need some time to digest it.

o *"Let's talk about the pros and cons of stimulants. This is the primary treatment for ADHD. I am obligated to tell you about this even though I understand your situation and that you don't want it. For ADHD the principal treatment is medication. Let me finish my obligation here, and then we can get back to the task at hand and talk about what else can help."*

—Steve Hughes, Ph.D.

Addressing stimulants in the context of comorbid learning disability

o "*I think medication helps certain kids more than others. Because of that, I have the reputation of having a balanced view. But for certain kids, I really see it will help. Your child has ADHD and a comorbid dyslexia. It turns out that unless you treat the attention piece, the therapy is not very useful for treating the reading problem. Sam is young, I am really glad I saw him now. If he was 14 or 15, we would have a very different conversation. If you are going to need to pay attention at any time during your academic career—it would be the first, second, and third grades, because you are learning the foundational skills for everything else that you'll be required to do in school. If you are going to go the medication route at any time, this may be the best time for him.*"

—*Bill MacAllister, Ph.D.*

He happens to have the only problem we have a pill for: talking to parents about stimulants

o *Your child happens to have the only problem that we have a pill for. We have memory pills but don't use them with kids. We don't have any pills for reading problems or language issues. We do have pills, though, for hyperactivity and they tend to work really well.*"

—*Bill MacAllister, Ph.D.*

What are the side effects of not using stimulants?

o "*You are right, there may be side effects to using the medication that are subtle that we aren't aware of, or are hard to scientifically measure. But let's think about it this way. What are the side effects of not using the medication that we know about? The attention problem continues to get in the way of John being able to maximally benefit from the reading instruction. It will be less likely that he can catch up to the other children. Remaining behind in reading is a very significant side effect—not a subtle unknown, possible side effect, but a huge, known, and very disruptive side effect of not using the medication. We can't guarantee that the medication will be a home run. But if it could take some of the attention problems off the table, it would be well worth it.*"

—*Karen Postal, Ph.D.*

I don't have a horse in this race metaphor for medication

o "*I'm a psychologist. Once my role is over, I don't prescribe. I have no benefits from pharmaceutical companies. I have no horse in this race.*"

—*Bill MacAllister, Ph.D.*

Why is the brain less important than the heart metaphor for medication

o *"If you have heart disease—would you take the medication? Yes! And if you had diabetes, would you take insulin? Yes! So tell me why you won't take medicine for your brain. Why is the brain less important then your heart?"*

— *Cheryl Weinstein, Ph.D.*

Computer electrical chord metaphor for stimulants

Sometimes parents worry that their child will feel they are defective if they "have" to take medication. Helping them and the child understand that the medication doesn't make their brain "smarter," but that it just lets them "use their brain" can be a helpful way to make them more comfortable with the idea of a stimulant.

o *"Let's pretend your brain is a computer"* (or an iPad, or whatever the latest "tricked out" technology is). *"It's a top of the line, comes with all the bells and whistles type of computer. I've downloaded every single program (or app) that you can possibly want. Well, that computer is worthless without the electrical cord (or battery). A stimulant medication doesn't make the computer better, it just helps it to run more effectively—it 'plugs your brain in.'"*

— *Kira Armstrong, Ph.D.*

Radio channel metaphor for stimulant medication

Sometimes parents are worried that medication will change their child—turn them into zombies, or maybe the medication will take away their creativity.

o *"I like to use an 'old-fashioned radio' to explain how medication should work for children with ADHD. You know how sometimes the radio station may be kind of 'fuzzy' or there may be too much static? The medication should help to tune in the radio station (in other words, it should help your child to focus better and show off all of his strengths). But it should not change the channel. If the medication makes your child act differently (in a negative way), if it changes his personality, then it's the wrong medication or the wrong dosage, and you should consult with your prescriber to see if there is a better option."*

— *Kira Armstrong, Ph.D.*

Double-blind trial for kids with stimulants

For parents who are concerned about medication effects, I offer the parents a four-week double-blind placebo trial that includes parent and teacher ratings, classroom observation, and a one-hour battery of repeatable executive measures, assessing the impacts of a randomized placebo, low-dose, and high-dose intervention. This can help convince even the stalwart opponent.

o *"I will be blind, Joey will be blind, the teachers will be blind, and even the gradu-ate assistants testing or observing Joey will be blind. Then you all can make an informed decision of whether medication is a good choice for Joey."*

—*James Brad Hale, Ph.D.*

Following children during stimulant trials

Reminding the family of your expertise and your willingness to be there to help make sure things turn out well often allows them to accept medication recom-mendations. You are not just being optimistic; if you are on the job, you are let-ting them know that you are there for them and their child will not spin out of control.

o *"The good news is—we're on the team. One of the things that we do is make sure that we go about the medication process properly. One of the great things about neuropsychologists is that we have an amazing array of tools at our disposal to help physicians understand the effects of medication and even engage in a titration process with them. I am willing to be responsible with you for whatever happens with your child. So here's what I want you to know. I am on the team, and I will not let this spin out of control. I've done this quite a bit and I will make sure that if we do medication, Billy will get better and not be a zombie. We will find the effective dose and I will help with that."*

—*James Brad Hale, Ph.D.*

Sometimes parents are ready to admit that their child may need some kind of medical inter-vention, but they are still wary about medication. In these instances they often seek out "nat-ural" treatment methods or scour the Internet to find other treatment options.

Rattlesnake toxin metaphor for alternative treatments

Parents often have a false sense of security about "natural remedies" just because they are not "medication."

o *"Just because a product is 'natural' doesn't mean it is safe. After all, rattlesnake toxin is 'natural' too."*

—*Kira Armstrong, Ph.D.*

Niagara falls metaphor for internet overload

o *"If you go on the Internet, you're going to find a whole bunch of scary stuff. Going to the Internet for information is like going to Niagara Falls for a glass of water. You're going to get some water. You're gonna get a whole bunch of stuff that you didn't intend to get. A lot of it is untrue."*

—*Bill MacAllister, Ph.D.*

ANXIETY AND ADHD

ADHD and anxiety disorders are frequently comorbid, in part because of the involvement of the prefrontal cortex in mediating both attention and emotional regulation. There is often a chicken and egg dilemma, when the presence of attention problems creates reality-based free-floating anxiety, which in turns dampens attention capacity. Depending on the clinical presentation, emphasis may be placed on treating one or the other first, or both at once. Patients and families frequently resonate with the idea that treating ADHD results in a reduction of anxiety, because there is less to be anxious about.

Children who have ADHD and an anxiety disorder often present with conflicting personality characteristics. When they are in their comfort zone they may be inattentive, dysregulated, and hyperactive, but when they are in a setting where they may worry about the possibility of negative evaluation (e.g., school), they may be especially quiet, eager to please, and will at least appear to be attentive. Similarly, at times they may work with at an especially slow rate in an attempt to reduce impulsive errors, but at other times they will work too quickly out of a need to "just get it done." I like to explain to parents:

> o *"This seemingly conflicting presentation is often seen in children who have both ADHD and an anxious temperament"* (or anxiety disorder). *"It is best understood by thinking of these characteristics as two sides of the same coin: your child's performance based anxieties and impulsive/careless behaviors are each an intrinsic part of who he is, but they are never present at the same moment."*
>
> —*Kira Armstrong, Ph.D.*

This helps families understand the connections between attention problems and mood issues. This also sets up a good rationale for why cognitive behavioral therapy (CBT) can be helpful.

> o *"Remember how we talked about the frontal lobe, and how it regulated attention? Well, it also regulates mood. Whenever you experience an emotion, there are two brain systems involved. The limbic system, also known as 'the lizard brain,' is this deep set of structures that produces waves of emotion. Like sadness or anger, or anxiety. The frontal lobe modulates these waves of emotion—softening them, or 'talking you down.' Here's a great example: road rage. You're driving along when suddenly another car cuts you off. Your limbic system sends out this great wave of anger, but your frontal lobe modulates—'Hey, that was a little old lady, she didn't mean to cut you off...' or, 'That guy in the truck has a gun rack, maybe you better calm down....'*
>
> *As the frontal lobe develops, it gets better and better at regulating emotions. Think about toddlers. They are great examples of little limbic systems running around without developed frontal lobes to modulate! Toddlers experience only waves of emotions. 'I'm happy! I'm crying! I'm screaming! I'm happy again!' As children grow, they get better at regulating their limbic emotional waves.*

"So just like Sandy's frontal system isn't able to direct her attention as well as it should for a third-grader, it also isn't modulating her emotions like it should for a kid her age. She tends to get overwhelmed with anxiety, or have a temper fit, or be overly giddy. Then she has ridden the wave and forgotten it, but everyone else in the room is still reeling. "CBT will help her frontal system regulate those limbic waves by practicing, ahead of time, good strategies for when she is nervous or mad, etc."

—Karen Postal, Ph.D.

o *"Jane is having so many 'oh, shoot!' kind of moments, or negative moments when adults are using a stern voice. Or she is forgetting things; she is always just waiting for the next shoe to drop. That's a hard place to be. She's also tired. She often doesn't get good sleep—and when she is trying, she is working harder than all other kids. When we give some relief to her, we will see a reduction in the anxiety."*

—Steven Guy, PhD.

Adhd and anxiety—treating ADHD is easier

o *"Look, if it's a matter of anxiety and ADHD, treating the ADHD is easier, and that may reduce the anxiety. It's an easier medicine, and you know the response right away."*

—Steven Guy, Ph.D.

BEHAVIORAL INTERVENTIONS AND COMPENSATORY STRATEGIES

Behavioral interventions and compensatory strategies are almost always a component of treatment for attention deficit disorder. The conundrum for adults is that if their executive function were intact enough to allow them to successfully engage in a new set of behavioral and compensatory strategies, they probably would not have been diagnosed in the first place. Inoculating patients against inevitable failures along the way may ultimately improve their compliance. The conundrum for children is that attention deficits have a genetic component, and their parents may not be able to implement the recommended system. For example, affected parents may be overwhelmed by the prospect of compensatory strategies. The first steps in the implementation of these strategies are identification, modeling, and "buy-in."

This helps teachers understand that small changes in the environment can help kids with who have ADHD:

o *"Having a little bit of unpredictability, but not too much, helps Jeremy have an optimal level of arousal. For example, when a teacher calls on people randomly, this increases anxiety and arousal, but just a little bit. The unpredictability essentially normalizes certain amounts of the cognitive dysfunction we see." (I always clarify that I am not talking about being disorganized as a teacher, but rather to planfully be a little unpredictable in order to keep children slightly on the edge of their seats.)*

—*E. Mark Mahone, Ph.D.*

ADHD Interventions—using music when doing homework

Often parents and children with ADHD get into heated conflicts about whether it is "okay" to listen to music while completing homework. Many parents think the child needs to work in an absolutely quiet room—but the child argues that they *need* music to work better. In these instances, parents see the music as another distraction that is further limiting their child's efficiency and productivity, even when the music may in fact be beneficial. Kids often love sitting in the room when I tell this to their parents—not only do they get to listen to music, they get to gloat over the fact that they were "right."

 ○ *"Although it may seem counterintuitive, if your child finds it useful to study while listening to music, he should be allowed to do it. Remember how we talked about the fact that ADHD is really an inability to control or modulate one's attention. Often children (and adults) with ADHD have difficulty regulating how hard they are focusing while working. Consequently they actually focus too hard (or, when it works for a family to use a car metaphor—"rev their engine too high"), "which leads them to 'burn out'—often before they are finished with their work. Listening to the radio helps them even out their attention, preventing them from hyperfocusing. This in turn lets them work for a longer period of time."*

  —*Kira Armstrong, Ph.D.*

 ○ *"Music during studying has been shown to help improve performance. But here's the catch—it can't be anything from your playlist! If it is in the background, no words, soft, relaxing ... then it helps to improve performance. But if they're GREAT songs, ones that grab your attention and have you singing along, then music won't help you study, it's going to distract you. Get your parents to help you put together a 'study playlist' of soft classical music."*

  —*Karen Postal, Ph.D.*

ACCEPTING THE DIAGNOSIS

The shadow of shame metaphor for accepting a child's diagnosis

The shadow of shame sometimes follows parents into the feedback sessions and blocks them from being able to accept the diagnosis or need for treatment, whether it's behavioral or medication interventions. They may feel an enormous amount of guilt for any genetically based disorder, including ADHD. The shadow of shame can become so big it creates defensiveness. The parent can't acknowledge the need for active intervention. "He's fine! He's fine! I was like that and I'm fine."

o *"That's great; you've developed fabulous coping strategies. You are here because your child hasn't learned them yet. What do we need to do to help him learn"?*
—*Jennifer Turek Queally, Ph.D.*

"This is not your fault. But it is your responsibility": helping children accept an ADHD diagnosis

When talking to kids about ADHD, parents frequently express concern that their child will start using the diagnosis of ADHD as an excuse. This pearl helps remove the blame while reinforcing their sense of responsibility.

o *"Let's be clear: this is not your fault. But it is your responsibility. What you will need to do, working with your parents, is figure out a way forward. And I want to let you know that others have been able to do this."*
—*Steve Hughes, Ph.D.*

EXPLAINING THE DIAGNOSTIC PROCESS

There is something magical about a folder of neuropsychological test scores. They are objective and feel "official" to parents and school districts. Providing feedback when children were not able to complete the testing because of attention or behavior difficulties can be challenging. Parents might feel that because all of the tests were not completed, a diagnosis cannot be determined. In some cases this might be true, but in many instances, the difficulty children have in our testing rooms reflects the difficulty they are having in their classrooms, and actually makes the diagnosis more certain. This section also addresses the situation when there is a significant disconnection between "rating scales" of parents and normal testing scores, or between the rating scales of parents and teachers.

This is useful when discussing test results of severely hyperactive kids who were climbing on the desk while they were being tested:

o *"Look, this hyperactivity cuts across the board. All of the tests capture attention in some way, but this is a microcosm of what happens in school. If this is what happens in school, he's only 'there' for a fraction of the time."*
—*Bill MacAllister, Ph.D.*

o *"He's delightful and curious. We got most of the testing done—let me tell you what we had to go through to get there. We finished one memory test under the table."*
—*Robin Hilsabeck, Ph.D.*

With many of the high SES kids in my practice, often the TOVA [Test of Variables of Attention] is the only thing a child falls down on.

o *"I'm testing your child in a highly structured, one-to-one environment, with not a lot of distractions. So if I can elicit any attention problems, it's reasonable to take that poor performance and assume that it would be even worse in a noisy classroom with 25 kids. Problems in my quiet environment will be amplified in the real world."*

—*John W. Kirk, Ph.D.*

Explaining a mismatch between rating scales and/or testing results

o *"When we do the testing, we understand that it's in a controlled environment; it's one to one. And that helps the child. It also helps us understand what they are capable of. If they are functioning differently outside that setting, then there's something about that other setting that contributes to their problems. This difference between scores also tells us that given the right circumstances, they can do better."*

—*Michael Westerveld, Ph.D.*

o *"Remember we talked about how the questionnaires were your chance to tell us how he functions in everyday life? So I am getting a lot of different messages about how he functions. The teacher didn't see much organization problems. But you are telling me that he has more organization problems than 99 percent of kids his age. What that tells me most about is your frustration with him not being able to do things on his own.*

—*Michael Westerveld, Ph.D.*

8 Somatoform Disorders

PROVIDING EFFECTIVE FEEDBACK—THAT is, delivering a message that will be heard constructively and acted upon—is particularly challenging with patients who have somatoform symptoms. Sometimes, clinicians may not even know they have a somatizing patient in the room until their "good news" of "no cognitive impairment" does not produce the relieved smile they were expecting. At other times, early in the initial clinical interview, it is clear that somatoform issues will be prominent. In either case, when working with this patient population, feedback can devolve into a tug of war between the clinician's desire to convince the patient they are well, and the patient's desire to convince the clinician that they are sick. Medical professionals and psychologists may find themselves trying to end this cycle by becoming increasingly authoritative: "This is my opinion. Take it or leave it," but when this happens, patients become dismissive, thinking, "Another doctor who doesn't get it."

Two common denominators emerge with the pearls in this chapter. The first is an emphasis on the clinician's respect for the patient's genuine experience of their symptoms. The second is the actively therapeutic stance taken to deliver their message; if the goal is to provide effective feedback with this population, a specific set of active, intentional, strategies, delivered with patience and skill, is required.

DEVELOPING EMPATHY AS A PROVIDER

Somatoform disorders: what suffering is honorable?

Something to think about: It takes a while to change your mindset, to see people with somatoform disorders as ones that are worth going to a level of effort to help. I went to a grand rounds presentation by a resident. It was a nightm`are. His theme was: "Somatoform patients are a pain. These people, we all know they can be 'challenging.'" While that is true enough, there was absolutely nothing constructive in this talk. He was just inviting people to validate those presumptions. Do you really believe these people are suffering? It gets back to the question "are they worthy of my time? because if they are putting me on, they are not worth my time." We all seem to be saying, "physical suffering is relevant and emotionally honorable. But this suffering over here, that the somatoform patients are experiencing, that suffering is 'weak.'"

This hierarchy of honorable suffering is clear in veteran populations. TBI is honorable. If something blows up near you, and it causes a brain injury, your suffering is honorable. PTSD is further down the list. While you went through something horrible, it's still psychological. Depression is caused by interpersonal weakness. That's what we "know." To say something is "somatoform" means you are either faking, or you are weak and not bearing up, and faking. —Greg Lamberty, Ph.D.

In giving feedback to other professionals regarding disability issues, sometimes our most important role is to help them understand the difference between malingering and somatoform disorder. Developing this awareness can make it easier for them to overlook some of the challenges these patients may present, and become more invested in their treatment.

Throwing the cane away metaphor for malingerers

○ *"I just wanted to explain how we have the ability to differentiate some of these things. With somatoform disorders, patients live the life they believe they have. They leave your office and live as an impaired person. The malingerer leaves your office and throws the cane away. They leave the office and live a normal life."*

—Sara J. Swanson, Ph.D.

ACKNOWLEDGING THE PATIENT'S SYMPTOMS

It is seldom productive to engage in an argument with patients about whether they have a disability or not. Similarly, focusing on the question of "organic vs. non-organic" is most often frankly counterproductive. Disability can be framed as not having the ability to carry out activities of daily living, and patients with somatoform disorders fit that definition, regardless of the etiology of their symptoms. An important first step in giving feedback to a patient with a somatoform disorder is to acknowledge the difficulties they are having, provide mirroring, and set up a collaborative stance. For example:

○ *"Wow! I can't believe how disruptive this has been for you. I can't imagine how frustrating it must be for you to not know what's going on, or to not be able to be the husband you want to be."*

—Beth Rush, Ph.D.

It helps to recap the patient's problems, so they are clear that you *did* hear them. For example, I was working with a woman who had migraines and falling spells. She developed physical symptoms and felt she couldn't drive, so she got people at church to drive her. She was a business owner, and she stopped working, but she was able to find household help that she felt she needed. And she felt cognitively impaired. All of the testing results were beautiful: high average across the board.

○ *"These are real problems. You are experiencing these cognitive concerns, but the tests show really good news. You scored really high on all the tests."*

—Sara J. Swanson, Ph.D.

INTRODUCING OTHER FACTORS, SUCH AS ROLE STRAIN, THAT AFFECT COGNITIVE EFFICIENCY

Many adults, particularly women, have taken on too many roles and get too little sleep, but expect their brains to continue to function flawlessly. A typical patient might have three kids under age six, work full time, and average five hours of sleep a night. Role strain can be introduced during the initial interview; clinicians might comment on the patient's daily stressors, "Wow! That makes *me* tired to hear about your typical day." In this process, clinicians foreshadow the discussion in feedback sessions.

"You can't sell your kids to science": explaining role strain

o *"You've got three kids, a full-time job, a marriage. Hearing your schedule made ME tired. You have what we call 'role strain.' You are working 40 hours, carpooling kids, helping with homework, managing a household, and a marriage. All of these pull on your time and attention making it very difficult to keep your attention on the thing you want to remember. I know there are too many critical things to realistically pare down. Obviously, you can't just quit your job or sell your children to science. But you can stop expecting your brain to work 100 percent of the time when it's under this much strain and overload. Rather than becoming distressed when you don't live up to an impossible expectation of 100 percent cognitive efficiency under all of this pressure, you should expect to have regular 'blips.' Give yourself a break when they happen."*

—*Karen Postal, Ph.D.*

Your brain has only so much energy metaphor for cognitive overload

o *"Your brain only has so much mental energy it can use per day"* (put my hands out as if trying to show how big something is). *"Right now, I would say that some of your energy is being taken away due to your level of anxiety, lack of sleep, and chronic pain."* (Move my hands closer together each time I say another contributing factor). *"As such, you only have this much energy to spend on everything you have to do today, including getting up and doing your daily tasks, going to school, going to work, taking care of your kids, etc. That's just not a lot of energy to do all of those things. This is likely contributing to being overwhelmed and feeling like you have no energy. Something has to give.*

So what typically happens is your brain goes on autopilot. You are still doing what you have to do but you are not truly engaged in the activity at hand. That is why you may lock your keys in your car or drive by your exit. It's not because you 'forgot,' but because your brain was focused on something else at the time and you were just going through the motions. Thinking-wise, what happens during this time is you may get the gist of a conversation but 'forget' the details. Not because you truly forgot but because you were not able to pay full attention in the first place.

For example, I can tell you how to get from here to 'X' and you can hear me say 'take highway Y,' but when you actually get there, you may not recall if I said 'east' or 'west,' and depending on which way you think I said, you could end up in two very different locations ... so all in all, you do NOT have a memory problem, you have a problem with attention in that you don't have enough energy to truly engage in the task at hand due to these other things such as chronic pain and lack of sleep snatching up the mental energy you would normally have. That is why you have been having some of the problems you were discussing with me earlier."

—*Andrea Zartman Ph.D.*

Praising overwhelmed patients

○ *"That's heroic! I couldn't do that. Plus a job, plus all the kids' sports. You're doing too much."*

—*Richard Naugle, Ph.D.*

○ *"It's really sometimes the strongest people who have what you have. They're trying to cope; they're trying to hold it all together. They're doing everything for everyone. And have to hold it all in. Eventually—no one could handle all that. And it comes out in physical symptoms. It's coming out in small ways with physical symptoms, and you're really experiencing those symptoms. You're really having pain, and really having episodes of forgetting. When we're dealing with difficult stress, our attention is focused on different things. So it really is difficult to encode memories. But when we get you in a quiet room and measure your memory—your memory system is great. So I know you will recover entirely from this."*

—*Sara J. Swanson, Ph.D.*

DISCUSSING THE MEANING OF NORMAL TEST RESULTS WHILE MAINTAINING A THERAPEUTIC RELATIONSHIP

A critical consideration when providing feedbacks to this population is to avoid equating normal neuropsychological performance with normal daily function; it is important to acknowledge that the patient with somatoform disorder is experiencing real symptoms, even if you are clear that the symptoms are not arising from a neurological problem.

○ *"The results of your exam show that your performances on testing were within normal limits, or where we'd expect, given your history and based on how we can predict your brain's level of functioning in good health. This data tells us about your brain's capacity when we try to control issues such as day-to-day distractions, fatigue, pain or headaches, or even stress related to the demands of the day. We try to assess you at your best, minimizing other issues that could impact your thinking. I appreciate that you are struggling day to day. This information helps us understand that your brain is capable of functioning well, but is probably struggling day to day because of issues other than brain damage. For example, I am concerned that your experience of pain and fatigue is distracting and limiting the amount of mental energy you have available to function optimally day to day. This information tells us your brain is capable of functioning well and also guides us to focus more intensively on the other issues that could be impacting your day-to-day cognitive struggles."*

—*Julie Bobholz, Ph.D.*

○ *"On formal testing, you're sitting here having to do certain tasks. Your brain is working as a normal person's brain would work. Somehow or another, when you're out in your daily life, something is preventing your brain from working as well as it is working here. And it's our job to try to help you figure out a way to identify what those issues are and how to overcome them."*

—*John Lucas, Ph.D.*

o *"I saw your cognitive inefficiency in my testing. It's not the kind that I typically see in patients that have something really wrong with their brain. And here's why. This was a really hard test, and you did really well on it. You couldn't have done so well if you had brain damage. And that's good news."*

—*Roberta F. White, Ph.D.*

Other factors that can affect memory

o *"Look, we are going to take a good look at your test data—and we will look hard for the factors that might be affecting your memory. Right now, these are the things I think are part of the problem. You're telling me you are averaging four or five hours of sleep a night. You have two demanding jobs"* (or, *"You are acting as a nurse and a mother," etc.) "When we are chronically sleep-deprived, parts of the brain responsible for online attention shut down. We go on autopilot. Things are getting done, but you're not necessarily paying attention. This affects memory. What your brain is telling you now, with these memory lapses, is 'I need more sleep.'"*

—*Cynthia Kubu, Ph.D.*

Hardware vs. Software metaphor for cognitive complaints

o *"How do we know what's going on with your brain? Well, we are going to look at your brain structures, like your memory system and language systems. Those are like a computer's hardware. We are also going to look at everything that is going on in your life, like stress, two jobs, not enough sleep, depression. This is like a computer's software. As you know from your computer at home, problems with the software can make the whole computer not work well. It is not always a hardware problem. Software is easy to patch ... hardware is tough. From this testing, it is clear that your problem is not a hardware problem."*

—*Susan McPherson, Ph.D.*

Memory can fail in everyday life

o *"Memory can fail in everyday life, but the problem won't be reflected in our testing. The flood of information we are all faced with every day may be distracting you. If you are distracted, you won't be paying attention; then it will feel like a memory problem."*

—*Munro Cullum, Ph.D.*

○ *"You know that happens to everyone. That happens to me. Maybe it happens to you more than it should. If you are looking for memory or other cognitive deficits, you will see them everywhere. Once you start looking for them, you won't be able to think of anything else. Be aware of that."*

—*Richard Naugle, Ph.D.*

Contextualizing the differences between the testing room and the real world invites patients to take responsibility for making changes in their day-to-day lives that will allow them to think better.

○ *"The good news is that on testing you did well. Now in here, the room was quiet and distraction-free. I kept you from being distracted. Out in the real world, you will have to keep yourself from being distracted. Let's talk about block scheduling, or a one-thing-at-a-time work process...."*

—*Susan McPherson, Ph.D.*

INTRODUCING THE ROLE OF STRESS AND EMOTIONS

After acknowledging the difficulty patients are experiencing, the next step is to introduce the mechanism that creates their symptoms. This conversation provides an important bridge between the symptoms they came in with and your recommendation that they seek psychotherapy. If the bridge is not compelling enough, patients will feel you are dismissing their symptoms by suggesting they "just need therapy," and may in turn dismiss the assessment process. It is critical to maintain a therapeutic alliance right up to the point where you get patients with somatoform disorders into treatment; if you allow them to dismiss you with, "I'm just going to find another doctor," then there is a good chance they will not get the treatment they need.

Kettle metaphor for stress

○ *"One thing that medicine does not know a lot about is the mind–body connection. Let me give you a way of thinking about the effect of stress on the body. Think about a kettle of water on a stove burner, with a lid tightly placed on top. The heat under the kettle is all the stressors in life—your job, kids, pain, your mother-in-law, finances.... When the water in the kettle gets overheated, the steam builds up, and has nowhere to go. Then the lid blows off. You know how that feels. That's when symptoms erupt. Pain gets bad, a migraine starts, and it's hard to concentrate. The built-up pressure has to come out somehow, and it comes out in symptoms.*

So instead of letting that steam build up, the key is to turn the heat down: like take more breaks during the day, go to a spa, practice being more assertive—asking others to do things for you. Sometimes, though, we don't have control over the heat. Our husband gets ill; there are layoffs at work and our job duties just doubled. Some things you can't control. So it's also important to learn how to take the lid off the kettle to let that steam escape. For example, exercise is a great way of releasing stress. Good sleep hygiene is another way of letting stress out. Another great technique is something called 'mindfulness training.' A psychologist can help you learn to let that steam out, so you don't get to the point of an explosion."

—Beth Rush, Ph.D.

Explaining the role of stress in cognitive complaints

I use the word "stress" a lot. It's kind of cool to have stress. I don't make it about their "psychological difficulties," or their "depression." Sometimes the stressors are obvious; sometimes the stressors are more subtle. The goal in feedback is to take the onus of the illness away from the patient and tell them it is caused by external factors. And then to tell them that they can learn to control those external stressors. The whole point of the somatoform symptoms in the first place is pursuing exculpation for pending failure. In men, it's frequently work-related. In women, it's often due to relationships.

> o *"I know this is probably being caused by stress. I can see one or two things that are stressors, but different people find different things stressful, and I'm not sure necessarily that I have a full understanding of what might be operating as a stressor for you. The funny thing about this type of stress-related problem is that the person experiencing the symptoms doesn't know either. That's why they have the physical symptom. You know, people who maintain a 'stiff upper lip about things' tend to have these symptoms, because they don't attend to stress when they should. They just sweep it under the carpet. But sooner or later it will come back to get you. For some people it's physical symptoms. For other people it's cognitive. You've been experiencing cognitive symptoms. But your testing showed that objectively you do better than most people your age. This is how I know your day-to-day symptoms are caused by stress."*
>
> *—Christopher Randolph, Ph.D.*

Stress and the immune system

With conversion disorders or patients clinging to a sick role, it is sometimes best to join them in the assumption that something IS wrong with their bodies. The immune system then becomes a metaphor.

> o *"Stress can affect the immune system, and that can have wide-ranging effects on many parts of the body. What we need to address is how you can lower your level of stress, so that the effect on your immune system, and overall health is lessened.*
>
> *—Cynthia Kubu, Ph.D.*

Depression and cognition

I put a lot of faith in the symptoms patients bring to me. In the course of the evaluation I try to explain to them why they have those symptoms. Whether it is something cognitive or psychological, or situational—whatever it is, I work hard to try to understand, so I can explain why the patient is having the symptoms. I share many of my thoughts in the process of the evaluation. I work collaboratively. I don't want news to be jarring at the final consult. I use an educational approach as I telegraph the information:

- *"This is what depression can do. Sometimes it's hard to know if a memory problem results from a neurological process or if it is the downstream effect of psychological factors. Memory problems don't have to be the result of a cognitive deficit. This is why I have included psychological as well as cognitive tests in the evaluation. Depression, anxiety, and emotional trauma, in addition to lack of sleep"* (depending on history, throw things out that might be contributing), *"sometimes old childhood head injuries, hormonal issues, they can all contribute."*

—Linda Vincent, Psy.D.

Pain can be a distraction

- *"When you are focused on pain, it's difficult to focus on what people are telling you."*

—Robin Hilsabeck, Ph.D.

Institutional somatization

In the military, physical causes are preferred findings. Emotional reactions and diagnoses are considered signs of weakness. Individuals within the military institutional culture are actively encouraged to prefer physical symptoms. The feedback conversation, therefore, is more likely to be effective if the word "stress" is used, rather than depression or anxiety.

- *"Let's talk about how stress is affecting your headaches."*

—Laurie Ryan, Ph.D.

Ataques de nervios

Ataques de nervios is a common emotional construct in Latino communities. Using this phase may be more effective than using terms such as "stress" or "depression."

- *"You're talking a lot about ataque de nervios, and that might be related. Maybe you're feeling sad and overwhelmed. I wonder if we were to make you feel less sad and overwhelmed—whether that would make your memory problem better?"*

—Monica Rivera Mindt, Ph.D.

INTRODUCING INTERVENTIONS

After joining with patients and acknowledging their symptoms, explaining the connection between stress and the symptom-production, and noting how CBT and exercise can relieve stress and therefore lessen their symptoms, it is time to "close the deal." Many clinicians use gentle humor and some motivational techniques to help move patients toward action. It also helps to recognize, and when appropriate even acknowledge to the patient, that part of the problem is a lack of awareness about what stressors are affecting them, and why. Of course, you can't just tell the patient "Become aware!" Instead you want to help them buy into the notion of how and why therapy will be beneficial.

> o *"We just talked about how stress builds up, like steam in a kettle, and how exercise and CBT can help you take the lid off the kettle and reduce that stress so you don't end up with so many symptoms. But I don't want you to jump right into this. You tend to be an overdoer. Am I right? I don't want you to go overboard. Of course, some people wouldn't do this at all, because they might consider taking the time to exercise and learn CBT techniques selfish!"*
>
> —*Beth Rush, Ph.D.*

> o *"Does it feel like it's so much more effortful to do things?" ("Yes!") "Well, chronic pain sucks energy from your brain. Things seem mentally exhausting. We need to find you a coach that you can see once a week—this is time just for you, not taking care of anyone else. You deserve that—you are all about taking care of everyone else—this is for you. The goals for the coach are to help you improve your sleep and exercise, things that put energy back into your brain. Anxiety also sucks energy from your brain as well. The coach can help you with some techniques to reduce that anxiety drain on your brain."*
>
> —*Cynthia Kubu, Ph.D.*

> o *"Regardless of what's causing your symptoms, it has a consequence to you in your everyday life. What I would recommend is that you need to learn how to cope with the changes in your life that these symptoms have brought upon you. I would recommend you seek some counseling. I don't want to give you the impression that your problems are due to depression alone. But depression is a byproduct of what's going on with you. In order to optimize your ability to cope, you will need to address the depression."*
>
> —*John Lucas, Ph.D.*

Light switch metaphor for introducing therapy

> o *"I want the therapist to help you with your pain management. I can see you sitting here. When you get tense, your muscles get all tensed up. If I sat like this"* (hunched over) *"I would be in a lot of pain too. It doesn't make you a bad person. I could just tell you to relax, but it's not like a light switch that you can just snap on*

and off. I can tell you to snap out of it, but you need to learn to do it. It's a thing you can learn to do. That's where the therapist can help."

—Jacobus Donders, Ph.D.

Empowering women

When working with women, it's important to empower them. Talking about a "disability" might not be the way to go.

○ *"Let's figure out how to use your strengths and cut your losses. We all get so caught up in worrying about makeup and hair. Let's take care of that brain. You can be empowered. Look at what you've done with your life!"*

—Cheryl Weinstein

Bolster your frontal lobe metaphor for therapeutic intervention

This helps create a new internal voice for somatoform patients, a new way of thinking about themselves. And because it uses a medical model, it is often easier for them to hear.

○ *"No one is walking in your shoes. It's really hard. We need to empower that frontal lobe by exercise, and good sleep, and use of structure; if your frontal lobe is fuzzy from decreased sleep or lack of exercise, then it will affect everything else in your day: your memory, energy level, even your ability to cope with pain. We have got to empower that frontal lobe to control negative affect from below. Your frontal lobe is getting hits. It's getting such rich information coming back and forward. But if you haven't slept, your frontal lobe can't handle it. You will get off track, and we'll have to figure out how to get right back on it.*

This goes back to the concept of Neuropsychology 101. Empower the frontal lobe; it's really about empowering yourself."

—Cheryl Weinstein, Ph.D.

Managing anxiety in rehab settings

○ *(For a somatically over-focused individual): "You're a person who tends to be very sensitive to changes in your body. Sometimes when people are upset or distraught, they react in different ways to that distress. You are someone whose stress comes out in a bodily reaction. For example, if you are sitting in an environment and you are feeling anxious, have you ever noticed your stomach feels tight, you clench your hands, and you breathe heavily? You might find you are experiencing that anxiety in a physical way. One of the things we want to do in rehab is to help you experience that anxiety in a way that it doesn't come out in a bodily problem. We will help you manage that anxiety, so you know when those anxiety signs are coming earlier on so they don't get in the way. We will also work with the rehab team to make sure that when that anxiety comes on we can deal with it right there and then, so it doesn't develop into a longer-term issue."*

—*Robin Hanks, Ph.D.*

Don't crush their soul metaphor for introducing therapy

Occasionally, when the patient is early in the development of the somatoform process, you might be able to suggest something that they will not find offensive. You will be the person who spent an hour talking about these things in a way that wasn't dismissing and soul-crushing to them. In the context of that warm feeling, if you can insert some suggestion for therapy, I am hopeful or naive enough to feel that this is a victory. Some might find meditation less "crazy" than CBT. There is even a grant-funded research program where they are giving trauma patients hatha yoga. The acceptance piece of yoga seems to help—just to get to a point where you put all of that negative, evaluative, "awful" stuff away for the moment. There's no psychobabble, it's physical, and patients can walk away saying, "I don't have to talk about my feelings to a shrink."

o *"A good exercise program can often help." (This is often met with, "Done that! That didn't work … that didn't work either"). "You also might want to consider yoga. With yoga, we seem to just feel better. It's not clear how. And it really doesn't matter how it works if people have less headaches. There are a lot of approaches now that bring forward this concept of mindfulness."*

—*Greg Lamberty, Ph.D.*

Psychotherapy changes your brain

One method of circumventing defensiveness and joining with the patients' conviction that the problem is physical, is to focus on the issue of how psychotherapy effects are physically mediated in the brain.

o *"We now know that any therapy that changes your behavior is working because it is changing your brain. It's the only way it can work. We are now learning the mechanisms of how the brain gets changed. And thus therapies are being more and more centered on brain-relevant mechanisms. We are learning about how the brain plastic changes underlie the effects of psychotherapies. We still don't have good enough knowledge of how the brain mediates these effects to give a clear prescription. A lot of the success will be dependent on finding the right person to be your therapist. It makes a big difference how that relationship evolves."*

—*Robert M. Bilder, Ph.D.*

Introducing cognitive pacing

There is a really interesting group of people with somatoform disorders who are overachievers. These people work *really, really* hard, and then something happens to them. They get sick, or have an orthopedic injury. They get time off, and they realize, "Oh my God, I spend my whole life going at top speed. Isn't this a great relief?!" Of course, any time anyone takes time off and then goes back to work, they're not as efficient. This group of patients misinterprets this decrease in efficiency as evidence of brain damage. Feedback becomes an opportunity to convince them to return to work in small bits so they can return to a comfortable place.

○ *"It's important that you start back to work and daily activities slowly. You know, don't even think about multi-tasking right now. Don't even think about working for three hours without a break. Don't even think about going back to work and school right now. Take it a little bit at a time. Tackle only one task at a time, and do that in a distraction-free environment. Don't even try to listen to the radio while working."*

—*Roberta F. White, Ph.D.*

FRAMING AN UNKNOWABLE MEDICAL ISSUE

Some patients are very invested in the sick role, and resist hearing that their cognitive problems are associated with a lack of sleep or some lifestyle issue. At times, agreeing that there may be an as-yet-unknown physical issue can allow them to feel heard, and "drop the rope" in the tug of war they typically engage in with their healthcare professionals.

○ *"Something else may be going on in your brain that we don't know about. But we do know about these issues, which are contributing to your day-to-day problem with memory, and we need to address them...."*

—*John Lucas, Ph.D.*

○ *"You know, our tests don't test for all the medical problems. It's possible that there are some issues going on that doctors just don't have tests for. But we see something on the personality testing that suggests you need help coping with all the medical problems that you are experiencing, with what you are going through."*

—*Sara J. Swanson, Ph.D.*

○ *"I can't tell you why, in your case, anxiety or nervousness causes pain in your shoulders. We are not sure how these things work. There are very complicated relationships between anxiety and the symptoms you are experiencing. So we want you to see a PT [physical therapist] or OT [occupational therapist] as well as a psychologist."*

—*Greg Lamberty, Ph.D.*

o *"Either you have a high stress level or your body is set to respond to stress below your level of awareness. This may be how you are physically built. You may be vulnerable to physical reactions in times of stress. Counseling can help with this."*

—*Gregory Lee, Ph.D.*

NORMALIZING SOMATIZATION

Sharing our own somatoform experiences helps normalize the process to patients. It's hard to dismiss the idea that there is a connection between their stress and physical symptoms as "just being called crazy" when their neuropsychologist is saying, "Yeah, this happens to me, too.…"

o *"When I get a migraine, inevitably, I stop and think, 'Oh! Yeah! I'm really stressed out.' It typically takes me getting a major headache to realize how stressed I am. Some of us just tend to experience stress directly in our bodies."*

—*Karen Postal, Ph.D.*

o *"I have migraines when my stress level is high. But my best example is when I was just about to turn 40. I was sitting in a meeting, and I had excruciating pain in my shoulders, and numbness in my hands. I had been working with a neurology group for years. And everything in the world pointed to me having MS [multiple sclerosis]. It doesn't have to be that obvious. But thankfully sometimes it is. And after my birthday, my 'exacerbation' went away! So even I have had this."*

—*Greg Lamberty, Ph.D.*

CREATING AN "OUT"

With somatoform symptoms, the feedback session is an excellent forum for creating a narrative about a path out of the symptoms. In this sense, feedback can play out like an Eriksonian story. Feedback creates an opportunity to provide an exculpatory "out"—some factor that one has no control over, like stress. The take-home message: the patient does not need to feel bad about "failing."

The focus of this message is externalization of the cause: stress. The symptoms are stress's fault, a mechanism they have no control over. It's not their fault. And it's not all in their head.

o *"There's a notion that stress affects your body, and causes your body to create symptoms that you can't control. With proper treatment, we can teach you to control those things."*

—*Christopher Randolph, Ph.D.*

The focus of this message is a suggestion that once a patient knows about the mechanism of the somatic symptom, he or she will naturally leave it behind.

I had a case in which a young woman who was undergoing a procedure for stomach complaints was given Versed. When she came out of the procedure, she couldn't remember anything from her whole life; she had complete amnesia. This was accompanied by "*la belle indifference*." She was eager to go back to school. Her presentation was cheerful; she couldn't care less. The back-story was that she had a lot of social difficulty at school in the last year. She had seen a psychologist and had developed all sorts of physical symptoms, including headaches. Now amnesia emerged and she was happy-go-lucky. In these situations, it is important to express certainty to patients and their families, to leave no wiggle room that it might be physical.

o *"Look, I know exactly what is going on with you" (leave no room for doubt). "Stress has been causing these physical symptoms. The Versed created a temporary amnesia that your subconscious identified as useful. Your subconscious took over and extended this over your life, so you became free of all the stressors that had been plaguing you. You couldn't even remember those schoolmates who had been giving you trouble. This is totally treatable. In fact, just knowing this will cause your memory to come back. And this is how it will go. You will return to school, and you will need to start psychotherapy treatment for the transition. I have some recommendations" (x-y-z therapist). Parents: "We liked that last therapist!" The girl (who to this point has been unable to remember any event in her life prior to receiving Versed) pipes up and says, "Is she the strawberry blonde with the fat ass? I'm not going back to her!" (Cured!).*

—*Christopher Randolph, Ph.D.*

9 Psychiatric Illness

SIGNIFICANT PRIMARY COGNITIVE impairment is often accompanied by mood or personality change. Conversely, primary mood or psychiatric disorders may also present with cognitive inefficiencies. For these reasons, neuropsychological assessments typically include an evaluation of mood, and the results of emotional evaluations have to be shared effectively with patients. Complicating this feedback is society's persistent bias against mood disorders and mental illness. Depending on a patient's ethnic, religious, and socio-economic background, this intolerance may be more or less pronounced. Although federal parity demands equal treatment of mental and physical illnesses, patients and families often have a strong, negative reaction to the news that a component, or the most significant component, of the patient's presentation is related to mood or psychiatric functioning. Finally, even when patients and their family are receptive to the diagnosis, it can still be challenging to explain *why* the patient is experiencing their particular cluster of difficulties.

Explaining schizophrenia and other psychiatric diseases

o *"We now understand that schizophrenia is a neurodevelopmental disorder. There is a difference in how the brain develops. The brain is wired in a different way, which makes it a little more difficult for you to process information in the same way most people do."*

—Bernice Marcopulos, Ph.D.

Undermining the diagnostic taxonomy with schizophrenia-like syndromes

I was involved in schizophrenia research for a long time, and I continue to get referrals for people with schizophrenia-like disorders. One of the things I do, much to consternation of my psychiatrist colleagues, is to assist patients in stepping outside of the tug-of-war with labels. By introducing the diagnostic issue in this way, I open the door to talk about their various cognitive functions. I really like to undermine the credibility of the diagnostic taxonomy à *la* DSM, and highlight individual experience instead.

o *"In your case, like everyone, you have a pattern of strengths and weaknesses. Your language skills are very good, but you are having some problems with your memory. I don't think that many of the diagnoses we have are particularly good at describing what is going on in your brain. These terms, like 'schizophrenia,' 'bipolar disorder,' 'ADHD'—these have all come out of trying to describe what doctors find out by talking to people, not necessarily what is going on in their brains. And we are still in a phase of development of the field where we are trying to find out what is going on in the brain.*

With people who have schizophrenia-like syndromes or bipolar disorder, there are no clear boundaries between these syndromes in terms of the real underlying biology. There are probably 1,000 genes that are critical to maintaining cognitive function and regulation of mood function. Some people are unlucky and get a combination of these things, which leads to brain function being easier to destabilize. The gene combination leads to problems with cognitive functions, like working memory, which makes you unable to keep many things in your mind and work on them like other people. Or the gene combination may prevent you from understanding the significance of things. So you might be in a situation where most people find it innocuous but you feel it has a lot of significance."

—Robert M. Bilder, Ph.D.

Feedback brochures

Often psychiatric inpatients have extreme deficits in attention. They may recall little of the feedback conversation. Therefore, our clinic came up with a brochure. Our process is to give feedback, then hand patients the brochure, which explains cognitive illness in mental illness.

o *"Thinking problems are part and parcel of any psychiatric illness, particularly schizophrenia. Here's how it affects you in everyday life."*

—Bernice Marcopulos, Ph.D.

ADDRESSING RESISTANCE TO FEEDBACK

Poor insight is common in psychiatric illness, and this can be exacerbated in a locked, inpatient setting due to a perception of coercion. Joining with the patient's perspective and giving them a sense of empowerment can help them be more receptive to the information you are attempting to share.

Clinicians can often empower patients by giving them choices. "You don't have to do this. If you want to say no, it's your right." This helps them feel more in control, like they have one little microcosm of choice and freedom. Sometimes this can allow patients to hear something, because they are not hunkered down and fighting.

o *"This is absolutely optional. You don't have to be here. This is a service that we offer. Since you spent the whole day with us, this will give you the opportunity to ask questions. I'll just go ahead and tell you briefly what the results were, but you don't have to stay if you don't want to."*

—Bernice Marcopulos, Ph.D.

o *"I know you don't think you have this problem. But what do those other people (who are wrong!) say? You know, this sort of fits with what your treatment team was concerned about." (If it doesn't fit: "Okay, what do you think might be going on?")*

—Bernice Marcopulos, Ph.D.

COPING WITH DELUSIONS AND HALLUCINATIONS

Attempting to directly contradict patients, or argue them out of delusions and hallucinations is rarely effective. A feedback session can be an opportunity to meet the patients where they are, educate them about neurological processes that may contribute to their (very real) perceptual experiences, and suggest some behavioral change without confrontation.

Never tell a patient their hallucinations are not real

○ *"Look, I don't see them or hear them. And I don't think a lot of other people do, but it must be upsetting to hear those voices. Let's talk about what's happening in the brain when we hear anything. We experience hearing something when the temporal lobe becomes active. This is the part of the brain hooked up to our ears. It's wired to detect sounds and then to make meaning out of sounds. What can happen sometimes is that there is activity in those brain regions—and it can occur even when the ear is not stimulated."*

—*Robert M. Bilder, Ph.D.*

Explaining extrasensory perception (ESP)

I participated in a project in which three patients in a small series all felt they had developed ESP or clairvoyance following their injury. For example, one woman said that she had a premonition that her very young daughter would injure her fingers in the door. Right after she had that thought, she felt pain in her own fingers. Then, sure enough, it happened to her daughter.

○ *"You know, in our own minds, we are always putting things in order. The truth of it is that our brain is holding in mind a lot of things at the same time. So when we recollect experiences, the order we put them in could be a little bit variable, particularly when you are emotionally upset—the order can be fluid. And we may get the feeling that this strong sense of empathy, and having the same feeling as your daughter, may have occurred earlier, rather than right after your daughter got hurt."*

—*Robert M. Bilder, Ph.D.*

DISCUSSING TREATMENT INTERVENTIONS

Affective recovery and wellness revolution

Something to think about: *The affective recovery and wellness revolution is a reframing of mental health care where patients are encouraged to take more responsibility for their illness. One purpose of feedback becomes educating patient so they understand how the disease works. The idea is to give them the tools, and empower them to manage their illness. The way to incorporate this into the feedback session* *is to focus on how the results suggest tools that will be helpful for them in managing their disease and day-to-day life, for example, using a day planner.*

—Bernice Marcopulos, Ph.D.

Good vicious cycle metaphor for therapy

o *"In the same way that your brain regulates your appetite or your blood pressure, it is also involved in regulating your mood states. Some people talk about approach and avoidance systems. We have in our brains these discrete, somewhat separable systems that will foster our going towards things, or withdrawing from things and getting further away from them. In some cases, people with mood disorders get stuck in a loop—they aren't getting very much positive reinforcement for approaching things, and they begin to withdraw more and more. So what's helpful is to try to build into your schedule some positive, reinforcing things, even if it seems hard to do at first. Getting out of that bad vicious cycle, and getting into a good vicious cycle, you'll find you are able to do more and more."*

—Robert M. Bilder, Ph.D.

Improving mood improves attention and memory

o *"We have a vast ability to learn new information, but limited attention ability. This is a problem, since we have to pay attention to learn. In general, our brains are pretty good at knowing what to pay attention to and what to ignore. For example, you don't pay attention to how your feet feel in your shoes or how your glasses feel on your nose. If you had to pay attention to all those little things, you wouldn't be able to pay attention to anything else, including listening to me now."*

Depression variation: *"So, you have this amount of attention"* (hold up hands to measure about a foot distance). *"But now you have depression, and you are focused on all those negative thoughts in your head. That reduces your attention"* (hold up hands closer together). *"This is the amount of attention you have left to learn new things. That's why it seems like your memory is so poor. With treatment for depression, you'll free up that attention again"* (hold up hands a foot apart), *"and you'll be able to learn new information like you did before."*

PTSD variation: *"You typically have this amount of attention"* (hold up hands to measure about a foot distance). *"I'm not paying attention to the noises outside the door, but you are; you've been trained to do that so you'll be safe. All that vigilance takes up the attention you would normally use for focusing on things you need to learn. That reduces your available attention"* (hold up hands closer together). *"This is the amount of attention you have left to learn new things. That's why it seems like your memory is so poor. With treatment for PTSD, you'll free up that attention again"* (hold up hands a foot apart), *"and you'll be able to learn new information like you did before."*

—Karin McCoy, Ph.D.

Offering hope to parents

Hope is so important for parents and kids with a psychiatric diagnosis.

○ *"One of the things that I want to communicate is that in my more than 25 years of clinical practice, I have seldom seen a kid who didn't somehow or other pull it together and make it. And I want you to know that. I know what you're going through now, believe me, I am a parent too. I want to try to help you. I am going to give you some constructive things that you can do at home, and that the school can do. And I will talk to her doctors, but I want you to know that she's going to make it. I know that because when I look at these scores, I see tremendous strength here … and I have seen it so many times before."*

—*Joel Morgan, Ph.D.*

SUBSTANCE ABUSE

Asking questions about how much alcohol patients drink weekly is typically part of the initial consultation. Discussing the impact of alcohol consumption typically takes place during the feedback session.

Quantifying alcohol use

Many patients pour large glasses of wine, or pour hard liquor directly from the bottle into their glass, and therefore tell themselves and others that they only have one or two drinks per night when in fact they are drinking the equivalent of four or five. A critical question to ask patients and their families at the initial interview, or during feedback is, "Do you use a jigger to measure the liquor, or do you judge the amount yourself?" Changing pouring behavior leads to a clear understanding of how much alcohol is being consumed. If the patient has a strong self-image as someone who "only drinks two a night," this can also actually reduce the amount of alcohol he or she is drinking.

○ *"Mr. Smith, last week we talked about alcohol. You told me you are having two gin and tonics each night, right? There are two reasons I ask everyone about how much alcohol they are drinking. The first is that after having a few drinks, people can get confused at night, particularly as they age. That may be playing a role in the symptoms your wife is noticing. Second, alcohol can be toxic to the memory system if enough is consumed over time. When we talked last week, though, you and your wife told me you just poured the gin in your glass, rather than measuring it with a jigger. We need to get a handle on how much alcohol you are actually drinking. Can we agree that you will use a jigger to measure over the next two weeks? Then I want you all to come back and let's sit down for another meeting to discuss whether we think alcohol might be playing a role." (Alternatively, this can be said during the initial interview, and reviewed at feedback).*

—*Karen Postal, Ph.D.*

Addressing substance-induced impairment

I give feedback to patients with alcohol issues while they are in an inpatient treatment center. The patients are often physicians. I always try to leave the door of hope open. Seventy-five to eighty-five percent are really unimpaired. The ones who are impaired—it's striking. I saw one physician who was practicing a week ago, and couldn't do Trails B.

o *"The testing suggests that your thinking is not as clear as it used to be and that you have some impairments that might interfere with your ability to practice medicine. You may need to consider other possibilities within medicine—practice settings that don't require rapid decision-making with patient care. There are other things you can do.*

You need to think about this. I know the last thing you want is to have some cognitive change you don't know about to affect your patient care. The last thing you would want would be to practice when you aren't able to serve your patients in the best way you can. But I'm not making the final decision. I will give this feedback to the team" (professional addictionologist, psychiatrists, etc.) *"This is a snapshot in time. I think you might need to go through another evaluation later to see how you are doing. These tests are not perfect predictors of something you have done your whole life. But again, when it's patient care...."*

—*Jim Irby, Ph.D.*

When people ask about whether their drug use caused cognitive deficits, we don't always have scientific evidence to answer the question. Of course, just because the research doesn't show that it's that big of a problem, it doesn't mean we want our kids eating paint chips.

o *"Well, I'm sure drugs didn't help you."*

—*Robert (Bob) Denney, Psy.D.*

UNCERTAIN PSYCHIATRIC DIAGNOSIS

o *One of my first patients had been sharing some very strange things, and he had an unusual MMPI, but it was hard to figure out what was going on with him. In the feedback session, I confronted him with this: "I don't know what's going on with you, but I feel you have some sort of secret or issue that I don't know about" (then he revealed that he had been assaulting kids on the beach).*

—*Roberta F. White, Ph.D.*

10 Learning Disorders and Developmental Disability

(countinued)

FEEDBACK SESSIONS FOR learning disabilities and developmental disorders are frequently highly emotionally charged. Parents may have differing views, as will other members of the extended family, about the origin(s) of their child's difficulties. There may be conflicts between parents and their child, who might have given up, as well as conflicts with the school to obtain services. Parents often sit with fears for their child's future, and may be grieving the loss of an experience of parenting a typically developing child. In this context, sharing results of the neuropsychological assessment is a delicate balance between offering clarity, creating room for multiple perspectives, and preserving hope. Although adults with learning disorders bring their own unique issues to the table, the majority of the pearls shared with us were specifically related to children. Still, many of these metaphors can be expanded to "fit" an adult patient.

DISCLOSING IQ

The same IQ score can have vastly different meanings, depending on the expectations of the patient and/or the child's parent(s). Highly educated, driven parents might become tearful hearing their child is "only" high average, whereas a couple with a developmentally delayed child might take a borderline IQ as a sign of progress. Misunderstandings relating to IQ ranges are also common, with some parents believing they were measured in the "200's" as children. Beginning the discussion of a patient's intellect, therefore, with an explanation of IQ as a construct and a framework for understanding the scores, can help avoid confusion and distress.

Explaining IQ

○ *"Okay, before we talk about the numbers, I think it's very important that you understand some things about IQ. A lot of times people come in and they have this idea—because that's the way it's portrayed on TV or the internet, or in books— that IQ is a trait that you are born with, and whatever you are born with is what it's going to be. And it doesn't change and there's nothing you can do about it. Nothing can be further from the truth."* (I then go through factors that affect development of IQ and IQ testing). *"So what we have is a snapshot in time, how your child is functioning today. Sometimes we think this is a good representation of how he does in relationship to his peers in the classroom, and sometimes we think it's not. And if not, I'll tell you why I think it's not."*

—*Michael Westerveld, Ph.D.*

Reassuring parents about average intellect

Depending on the parents, the term *average* can sometimes be a negative descriptor. This phrase helps put "average" in better perspective.

○ *"She has nice, well-developed, average intellect. This score means her intellectual development is right where it should be."*

—*Karen Postal, Ph.D.*

o *"You're lucky. Yes, she's average, just like most people are. There's nothing to hold her back here from whatever she wants to do. Most people are average. You don't need genius to be happy and healthy."*

—Laurie Ryan, Ph.D.

Helping parents recalibrate expectations

This is a message I give to high-powered parents who need their kids to be gifted, and are disappointed with average or even high average scores:

o *"You could have him in all these extra classes, and tutoring, and all that. And he may get in" [to that advanced school]. "But he's 12, and what he'd really like to do is go to the football game at the high school, and play some video games. He's going to do great, and be able to do anything he wants to do. Are you putting too much pressure on now?"*

—Christopher J. Nicholls, Ph.D.

INTELLECTUAL DISABILITY/MENTAL RETARDATION (MR)

When parents hear the terms *mental retardation* (MR) or *intellectual disability* for the first time, it is important to allow space in the room for an emotional reaction. Clinicians can do this by literally stopping, and asking a question to invite parents to discuss their reaction. At times, the reaction may be anger and disbelief: parents may be out of touch with their child's skill set—expecting too little or too much, and they may not understand the developmental trajectory that can be expected for their child, given the developmental delay. At other times, parents recognize the diagnosis as a validation of their greatest concerns and fears.

Diagnosing mental retardation/intellectual disability

o *"So, we completed our testing and the findings suggest that your child qualifies for a diagnosis of mental retardation." (Then you stop. Maybe silence.) "What do you think about that? Is this something you considered?" (This opens the door for an emotional reaction, and it evolves from there into a conversation.)*

—John Beetar, Ph.D.

One time, I was giving feedback to young parents about their child who had MR. The father stood up, declared "I don't agree with you," and stormed out of the room. The mother said, "Keep on going, keep on going." I think it's a mistake, if you haven't been there, to say, "I understand what you are going through." I am sitting in relative comfort. I may be anxious about what's in front of me, but it's nothing like they are experiencing. I was a trainee the first time that I gave feedback that a child was MR. A week later, the dad wrote a thank-you note. People want to hear the truth, ultimately.

o *"I don't have children. And I am not sitting where you are sitting. In no way can I appreciate what you are feeling."*

—*John Beetar, Ph.D.*

Using personal experience

I will bring in my personal experience, which helps build some "street credibility." By sharing the information, I can convey to parents that I have an understanding of what they are going through, on an emotional level. I literally see patient's families' faces change.

o *"I have a little sister with Down syndrome."*

—*Bill MacAllister, Ph.D.*

Just as with the diagnosis of Alzheimer disease (see "Using the A Word" in Chapter 6) when clinicians use the words "mental retardation" can also vary.

Using The MR Label

I wouldn't diagnose a child under four with MR, even though I might know. In these cases I might use the term *global developmental delay*, which doesn't assume as much about the future. But, if the child is five and beyond, or has received at least one to two years of good educational or Early Intervention services, then I really want the parents to know that their child is somewhat cognitively limited. If the parent is either in denial about these limitations, or highly anxious, I might try to get them less focused on the future and get them to where he is functioning now. This leaves the future open for them, even if I know that things are not likely to change that much in terms of global delays. This might allow them to keep their defenses intact as far as facing their child's ultimate limitations and help them mobilize to immediate action. As the child gets older, the reality usually sinks in, and usually sooner rather than later.

o *"This is where your child is functioning right now. He is five years old and he's functioning at a 2.5-year-old level in this area, a three-year-old level at this," (and it's almost always the case that the Vineland agrees with the cognitive data). "So, this was pretty consistent, both what we saw in the office today and what you reported he does in every day life. It's all a pretty consistent picture that he's performing two years behind.*

So, we should try to focus on the present instead of the future. We just need to worry about where he is functioning right now. That is going to dictate what services he needs in the immediate future, and that's all we need to worry about. As time goes by, we'll get him the best we can get him, and the picture will become clearer."

—*Deborah Fein, Ph.D.*

I feel that it is important to use the term *mental retardation* with families. "Intellectual disability" is not in the DSM-IV.

> o *"I have to call it 'mental retardation' in order to make your child eligible for different services. That's the diagnostic criteria. Right now, Congress, the State of Massachusetts, some schools are trying hard not to use that term. And maybe in the next 10 years, we may not see the term. But for right now, we need this term, 'mental retardation,' to get the services. However, some schools might use the term 'intellectual disability' and they are talking about the same thing."*
> —Jennifer Turek Queally, Ph.D.

In Minnesota, there are different names for things depending on whether it is a medical diagnosis or educational eligibility category. I will spell this out to the family in the feedback session, and include it in the report. (Text of report):

> o *"Parents and families would refer to this as an Intellectual Disability. The medical diagnosis is moderate Mental Retardation, and the schools' eligibility category for special services is Developmental Cognitive Disorder."*
> —Karen Wills, Ph.D.

If children are at a 71 IQ and they are six years old, I will have this talk with the parents. Just as, if some one had a leukoctye count of 9,999, you would say they are one point away from high-risk. No other medical profession would *not* have this talk. But it seems like a lot of psychologists might not discuss MR with parents until the child's score is 69.

> o *"You know what, we are on this developmental trajectory"* (image of an upward trajectory.) *"If we don't keep that line up close to the line of the other children, and it slips a little lower, then he will meet the criteria for mental retardation at some point in the future. Let's talk about what that means."*
> —Jennifer Turek Queally, Ph.D.

The problem with using "delayed" instead of the MR label

It surprises me all the time how often other professionals continue to tell parents of school-aged children, "Your child is delayed." I see kids where professionals have clear information that the child is performing poorly—both adaptively and cognitively, and this is not a recent decline that may be reversible. This is a problem because the term *delayed* implies they're going to get there eventually, they're just "late"; they're going to get to the party, they're just tardy. But this is misleading, and I often feel like the bad guy sitting with the parents saying, "Your child's developmental progress at this point is consistent with mental retardation." They're surprised: often commenting, "But I thought he was delayed!"

I've learned not to back away from the diagnosis. Early in my career, I would back off from the diagnosis when the child's functioning fell in a gray area. I would talk myself out of it, because the parents or what they might say would sway me out of making the diagnosis. But I've been at this same place with the same kids year after year, who carry this "delayed" label—and the stories—the kids are getting worse, and the parents will say, "I just know if we can clean up the meds, things are going to be different." Even if we get these things under control, this child is not going to be operating at a level that is within even a broad margin of the typical range. At that point, I think you really have to make the diagnosis. I've also had that awkward experience of *not* making the diagnosis, and now years later I see the kid again—they're not that different, but now I'm making the diagnosis. And I have to reconcile with myself and with the family, why didn't I make that diagnosis earlier? What if that kid doesn't come back to you until they're 18 years old and one month [and they're now not eligible for disability services]? I err on the side of giving it now, I don't back off from it, and I try not to make it a big, heavy thing.

    o *I'll tell parents, "This doesn't change who your child is at all. This is just a combination of your child's adaptive function and intellectual function being lower than the typical group. This is consistent with your child's trajectory over time—the gap between your child and his peers has widened over time. This diagnosis is helpful in understanding your child's prognosis, and identifying them as a person who is in need of a certain type or level of service. It's my responsibility to document that for your child."*

                                                    —*Katrina Boyer, Ph.D.*

EXPLAINING INTELLECTUAL DISABILITY/MENTAL RETARDATION

    o *"There's a certain cutoff that determines how many services different agencies will provide. There's a line that everyone has agreed to use—the state, psychologists, schools, etc. If you score above the line you get a certain level of services, because you are higher-functioning. And if you score below, you get more services, because everyone has agreed that you need more. It's an arbitrary line because there isn't a lot of difference between 69 and 71."* (Most parents understand where she is going at this point). *"In order to meet criteria, to determine what level of services your child needs, we have to determine if he meets criteria for mental retardation. Which has horrible social connotations, but mental retardation does not mean all the things you heard in middle school. What it means is that mental development has been retarded or slowed. That's where the term came from. It means that he's still developing, but at a slower rate. Because your child scored below 70 on both the IQ and adaptive measure, he now has the option of becoming eligible for more services."*

                                       —*Jennifer Turek Queally, Ph.D.*

Parents may ask, so if we come back next year, will his IQ be normal?

    o *"He will continue to develop. He won't be the same child he is today. But his trajectory is different than other children's."*

                                           —*Deborah Waber, Ph.D.*

Normalizing declining scores

Helping parents understand development over time with MR, I draw a chart with skills as one axis and time as another.

o *"Hypothetically, development goes like this. It's a little bit bumpy, as anyone with children knows. If we start out on the developmental track, and then we have a big impact, like cancer treatment—that stagnates development for a while. And then we get back on the developmental track, then this difference in distance will be maintained over time, while the child continues to develop. If something happens here that changes the brain, we might not be able to keep the original trajectory. We may not be able to learn as quickly, and then the gap gets bigger. Even though we might start out really close to the other kids, as time goes on and tasks get more challenging, the gap will get bigger. Our goal is to keep the gap as small as possible with therapies and interventions. They are going to keep learning, but at a slower pace. We will probably have to choose certain things to focus on, because the child won't be able to learn everything."*

—*Jennifer Turek Queally, Ph.D.*

o *"This is what we might expect in the future. You may see these scores go down. It doesn't mean your child's skills are going backwards, it just means that he is not developing at the same rate as his same-age peers. Don't worry about the scores. Just keep moving forward."*

—*Bill MacAllister, Ph.D.*

Discussing the meaning of mr or intellectual disability

o *"Given where these scores are, this is the type of things we can expect."* (If they are really low,) *"It's really early in the course here, but in general, this is not the type of kid who you would expect to be able to live independently—to cook for themselves, to clean for themselves...."*

—*Bill MacAllister, Ph.D.*

Assessing the parents' understanding of their child's limitations

Clinicians don't always know whether parents understand that their child has an intellectual disability. It can be helpful during feedback to begin by assessing what they know about their child's abilities.

o *"On a developmental level, what year do you think she is?"*

—*Bill MacAllister, Ph.D.*

HELPING FAMILIES DEFINE THEIR CHILD'S STRENGTHS

o *"Although the academic arena is probably not going to be one where Sally will distinguish herself, she has many other strengths that will serve her very well in life … for example, she is very social, enthusiastic, and loves to cook. At this time, your most important job will be to make sure you and her teachers keep their expectations at a level that will allow Sally to continue being the social, happy girl she now is."*

—*Ketty Patiño González, Ph.D.*

Good enough for life metaphor for defining strengths

o *"If you look at most of our neuropsychological data for children, for example, how many items you need for an average score on any of our tests. Initially the scores go up very rapidly, but they taper off in adolescence. What you can see is that around adolescence, after 11 or so, you don't have such a rapid gain. You hit a point where you get to an adult level of function at some point in adolescence. This is normal development. For a lot of developmental disorders, what happens is that you have a protracted trajectory. They have an early trajectory that's not so bad, but then the gap gets bigger, and their trajectory takes longer. So what happens after these guys over here hit their peak—these guys are still making slow and steady progress. Children with developmental disorders are still going to continue to develop, compared to themselves, even when other kids are at an adult level of performance. In other words it just extends the developmental framework. They don't need to finish high school at 17, or get into college right away. Or get a job right off the bat. Who cares if it takes an extra year to finish high school these days—especially if it makes everyone saner."*

—*E. Mark Mahone, Ph.D.*

CORRECTING MISUNDERSTANDINGS ABOUT A CHILD'S ABILITY LEVEL

Parents may overestimate their child's language abilities. Some say, "I know he doesn't talk much, but I know he understands everything we say." Then you test the child, and even though he's five, he's got a language comprehension of 18 months. Most parents really begin to understand when you show them the evidence.

o *"He could follow a one-step command, but as soon as we got to two-step commands, he really couldn't do it. He looks like he's understanding, because he's looking at you. He's very smart about picking up social cues, he's picking up on your facial expressions and your gestures, but if you actually test the words and the grammatical forms, he can't really understand without cues from the environment. Really his language ability is lower than you think. He understood these words, but not these words. So, he's pretty consistent in his own performance and that really suggests to me that he may be understanding your social cues, but he's not understanding your language. Rather, he understands what you want him to do. So if you want to help him, you have to simplify your language. You have to talk to him like you would talk to a much younger child."*

—Deborah Fein, Ph.D.

SEXUALITY

It's uncomfortable for any parent to think about or talk about their child's sexuality. This discomfort is often magnified in the context of developmental disability. Clinicians are not immune to our culture's discomfort with the topic, but it is very helpful for neuropsychologists to bring up sexuality—because parents may not know they can.

(I have this conversation for both boys and girls.) When a teenager has fine motor difficulties, the feedback conversation will often come around to the subject of sexuality.

There is nothing that leads me to believe that youth with motor and cognitive problems aren't as interested in sex as anyone else. It raises interesting questions. If you have a motor deficit, how do you masturbate? How do you assure that everyone has consented to sexual activity? Some of the youth we see are almost never left alone or unsupervised, and some might not have the motor capabilities for sexual exploration. As you can imagine, this can be very awkward to talk about. They are thinking about sexuality, but they don't have the means to explore it, even just on their own. Of course they want romantic relationships too, but that's a whole different issue.

We tend to focus our intervention and accommodation ideas on school-related issues, but we can be fairly oblivious of the barriers to other aspects of personal functioning that medical issues create. When discussing this in a feedback, a father once said, "You know, this kind of conversation is a great opportunity for us to think about how *we* are parenting this very complicated child, rather than focusing only on what the school is or is not doing."

o *"This is something ... I don't know if you are thinking about this,,please just tell me to shut up if you don't want to talk about this.... What about your kid's sexual life? How are they equipped to experience this aspect of life? It's difficult to talk about sex with a typically developing kid, but this is even harder. Most parents have the luxury of thinking, 'We don't want to know about it,' while sexual development occurs, a type of implicit 'don't ask, don't tell' agreement. That may not be a luxury that parents of medically involved kids have. Should you buy them an adaptive vibrator or a masturbation sleeve? It's difficult to know the right way to proceed, but it may require a more intentional and thoughtful approach."*

—Andrew Zabel, Ph.D.

Sexuality: this is not a morality issue

o *"Have you all talked to your child about masturbation? Are you comfortable talking to him about this? It's helpful to explain to the child that this is something that's okay to do, but they have to do it in their bedroom or their bathroom, they can't do it in front of other people. This is not a morality issue. This is a social acceptability issue. This will make them ostracized if they engage in these behaviors in the wrong setting."*

—*Deborah Fein, Ph.D.*

Sexuality: changing a lot of sheets lately?

o *"Doing a lot of laundry these days? How are you handling masturbation? Or public displays of sexuality?"*

—*Christopher J. Nicholls, Ph.D.*

LONG-TERM PLANNING FOR SEVERELY IMPAIRED CHILDREN

"What will my child be like when they grow up?" Some parents wonder if their child will be able to leave home at 18, while others may be more worried about "what will happen when we die?" After a diagnosis of significant developmental disability is disclosed, parents often turn to questions about the future. This question can be difficult to answer, especially in a single feedback session. In some clinics, neuropsychologists have the luxury of following children closely, sometimes multiple times a year. This gives them the opportunity to address these questions again and again. Even if you are practicing in a different setting, many of these pearls can help you to support parents as they work through their fears and goals for their child with special needs.

"This doesn't look good now, but because this hasn't been identified before, he's never gotten the help he really needs. We don't know what he will look like when he gets that help. From your child's perspective, school won't feel so bad—because he's in a situation that is more manageable—so you will probably see a nice change for the better."

—*Deborah Waber, Ph.D.*

Something to consider: When working with children with severe disabilities, neuropsychological testing and feedback sessions are not developed merely to establish patterns of deficit, but to establish patterns of capability and things that can be built upon.

The problem with very involved medical populations is that these children often don't achieve full independence in anything: in their mobility, their independent functioning, their living situation, etc. I think it's crucial to take a perspective of expanding independence rather than simply achieving independence, either through accommodation or modification. If the child can't unload the dishwasher, she might still be able to sort the silverware. She can still participate to her capacity.

—*Andrew Zabel, Ph.D.*

Reminding parents that most young adults are supervised in other settings can make the need for supervision after high school easier to process.

o *"High school students who go off to college are supervised by resident advisors in the dorms. High school students who go into the military are well-supervised in that setting too. Your child will leave home, and also go into a setting that's well supervised. This is similar to what other people do for a while when they leave the house."*

—*John Beetar, Ph.D.*

Fostering functional independence

Families may have difficulty shifting their children with disabilities into greater independence. "If only she would wake up on her own!"

o *"You are going to expend energy in your parenting—rather than spending it in an argument as you wake her up every morning, why not spend it rewarding her for using an alarm clock?"*

—*Andrew Zabel, Ph.D.*

Long-term planning: considering other family members

When discussing long-term plans for children with significant intellectual disabilities, denial is common. Parents might say, "We don't need to make any arrangements; his sister says she'll take care of him for the rest of his life" (even though the sister is only 14 at the time).

o *"Well, I would encourage you to still think about other options, because Sally is only 14 now. And while she loves her brother and expresses an interest—she may also want to go to college and pursue her own goals. So having another plan in place in case something like that happens is important."*

—*Jennifer Janusz, Psy.D.*

LEARNING DISABILITIES

The idea that a child has pockets of true deficit in the context of normal intellect is difficult for adults as well as children to fully comprehend. Many children have the conviction by the time they are assessed that their difficulty with, for example, reading means they are "dumb." Likewise, parents intuit their child's best cognitive abilities, and may feel that if only their child tried harder, or more, they could perform normally in the area of deficit. Whatever the underlying assumptions, the discussion is often emotionally charged, and may tap into intergenerational issues, due to genetic contributions to the disabilities. There may be a complex emotional history and unhelpful narratives about the relatives who had similar profiles. Parents may be listening to their child's results while engaging in reverie about their own, similar struggles during their childhood. Could this explain their learning problems? Maybe their own negative assumptions about their thinking abilities are not correct.

On the other hand, some parents may feel an overwhelming sense of guilt—"I should have *known* better! How could I have let him struggle for so long?!" Often this occurs even when parents have asked schools for help and assessments, only to be told that their child was "just fine." Just like in so many other clinical situations, presenting our findings and their implications clearly enough to convince families the problem is real, while assisting parents in holding their child's strengths in mind, is an art. So is helping them to let go of the guilt. The following analogies are elegant solutions to this dilemma.

o *"My results prove that you are a really smart kid. But, I'm betting that you don't always feel smart. Here's why...."*

—*Gail Grodzinsky*

o *"We all have strengths and weaknesses. We all have things we're good at and not good at, like artistic abilities. Your son has the same thing, but more exaggerated. He happens to have weaknesses in areas required for academic skills. If we lived in the South Seas Islands, and the goal was to learn to row a canoe to the next island, Johnny's strengths and weaknesses would not be considered a disability."*

—*Gerry Taylor, Ph.D.*

Explaining the impact of focal impairments on global functioning

o *"Given these two or three impairments are so severe, they serve to depress his overall ability. Your child is not able to marshal his resources and show what he is able to do. Using on our tests, in this structured environment, we are able to isolate these skills, and highlight his strengths. But in everyday life, like school, where people are required to put it all together, he is just unable to because of the impairments."*

—*John Beetar, Ph.D.*

Lighter fluid in a jaguar engine metaphor for reduced processing speed

When verbal and nonverbal intellectual skills are strong, but working memory and processing speed on intellectual testing is impaired, this is a helpful metaphor.

o *"Working memory and processing speed represent input and output. Your child has good thinking and reasoning skills; his verbal and nonverbal intellect are well developed. But his working memory and processing speed are relatively weak. It's like pouring lighter fluid in a Jaguar engine. The car will run, but not as well as it should."*

—Cynthia Levinson, Ph.D.

Clutch metaphor for automaticity

Everything we learn has a declarative component and a procedural component. They operate on separate trajectories, and we often lose sight of the procedural component, which is very important. Many children with developmental disorders have involvement of the basal ganglia and cerebellum, which are very important for procedural learning. So what we don't see in a lot of these children is the automatization of a lot of these skills.

o *"When you are learning a skill, you are activating more of your cortex. That's called 'declarative learning.' Then, when you become proficient in the skill, and it becomes over-learned, your brain uses less cortex. Then we call it an 'automatic skill.' Unless, if you have had something happen in your brain—in that case that switch to procedural automaticity doesn't happen so quickly.*

For example, consider basic things like writing—writing is something that has to be thought about. It's an active learning process for a long time. Or sound symbol relationships, or math facts. For children with developmental conditions—these tasks become automatic less quickly. The process stays declarative, and they have to think about it. And if they think about it while doing it, they develop all these bottlenecks. For example, when you first learn to drive a clutch, you have to think about every movement you make. You have to turn off the radio, put away your lunch, not talk. After a while, it becomes automatic. You don't have to think about it any more. You can turn on the radio, eat your lunch. That's great, until it starts to rain. When it's raining, you need to concentrate more. You have to turn off the radio."

—E. Mark Mahone, Ph.D.

Explaining the impact of visuomotor deficits

When speaking to parents and school teams—I try to relate testing performances to everyday life. People typically have trouble understanding visuomotor function.

o *"In school, this could mean that the child could have difficulty copying notes from chalkboard to notebook, or making graphs in algebra."*

—John Beetar, Ph.D.

Explaining dyslexia and language disorders

o *"Let me explain the four components needed for effective reading. To read, you need to take in, take apart, and put together the sounds that make up words.*

For example, you have to be able to hear the three sounds of the word Cat: kuh–a–tuh. If you can't do that when listening, you won't be able to do that when reading. Then you will be really slow when you are trying to sound out words. The next piece is rapid naming. We did that task where I asked you to name words within a time limit. You eventually got the word, but it took time. That's the second piece: after you have decoded the word, you have to make the connection in your brain with what it means. If you can't do that rapidly, that will also slow you down. The third piece is comprehending what you hear. If you have trouble understanding what you hear, you will have the same problem understanding what you read. That will slow you down, too. The final piece is 'span' for what you hear. You have trouble with your span, which means that what you take in now knocks out what you were just holding in your mind. If you are given too much information at once, then you will overload. This can affect you when you are listening, particularly if the information is complex, the speaker goes quickly, and you have to take notes! The same thing will happen when you are reading, because by the time you get to the end of the paragraph or sentence, you've lost what's at the beginning—so you have to go back and read it again."

—Robb Mapou Ph.D.

Many school assessments fail to recognize how kids are compensating for poor dorsal-stream functioning by using the ventral stream to read whole words. These children can't decode, and they can't do pseudoword reading to save their life. Many school psychologists will dismiss the problem given a child's average score, even though we know of the importance of early intervention for dorsal stream reading problems. We need to intervene now, while he still has average scores. Kids need both the dorsal and ventral streams to read well, and if they don't acquire these skills, comprehension will eventually decline as they recognize fewer and fewer words.

o *"There are two pathways to reading words. Read this" (gives parents a sentence with five or six words). "Did you sound out those words? No, because sounding out is the first step. Being able to look at the letters and decode—is the first stage in learning to read. The second stage is being able to transfer that to an automatic reading by sight. There is no way we can sound out the words and be any good at understanding what we read, or read reasonably quickly if we are sounding things out.*

This automatic sight word reading is something that we want to work toward: but it won't work forever in kids that can't sound words out too. That is because you can't memorize all the words you need to read. You have to be able to decode words too, and then link them to known words in memory.

Jon is in first grade and got an average score on a reading test, but he can't read pseudowords, he can't sound them out. His errors are meaningful sub-stitutions (like saying the word 'tried' for 'true'). The real problem is that in first and second grade, you can memorize enough words to read in the average range, because there aren't too many words to memorize. But by middle school you just can't memorize enough words by sight, so you need to decode the unknown words, and link them to your knowledge of words. If you can't decode, you will fall further and further behind, and you won't understand what you read, because you'll skip too many words, or guess wrong when you try to read them."

(Now show parents a sentence with college-level words.) "Did you have to sound some of these words out? How did you read the words?" (Parent: "When I read it, I started to sound them out, then I recognized the words.") "Well, Jon will need that skill, and right now he doesn't have that. He will need to be able to decode the words to link to his vocabulary memory."

—James Brad Hale, Ph.D.

Some children only decode; they have no sight word vocabulary. So their reading fluency will be very poor. Their higher-level comprehension will also go out the window, because their "working memory" is being used for decoding, not understanding.

o   *"If Johnny is using up all of his working memory for sounding out words, he won't be able to keep track of what the heck he is reading so he can understand it. Sometimes kids' working memory is so taxed by decoding that when we ask them what they have read, they don't have a clue."*

—James Brad Hale, Ph.D.

Foreign language metaphor for language impairment vs. Inattention

o   *"You're right, you have seen this, but it's not because he's inattentive. If you spoke to me in Russian, I would stare out the window, too."*

—Deborah Waber, Ph.D.

Language deficits with intact vocabulary

Parents often struggle to understand why language is impaired even when a child's vocabulary is good.

o   *"I gave your son a task where we asked him to define the word island. And he, like a lot of kids who are concrete with language said, 'You take a boat there! And there is sand! And there are umbrellas in your drinks!' All of that is true, and it all tells me about an island. But the most important part of island to know is that it is a hunk of land surrounded by water. If you child never ever gets to that part, he's not always communicating as effectively as he could be. And that's where I get worried. Actually having that fabulous vocabulary can be a risk factor.*

*Because others hear the vocabulary, and never understand that he has difficulty
with language."*

—Jennifer Turek Queally, Ph.D.

USING SPECIFIC TEST PERFORMANCES TO EXPLAIN DAILY DIFFICULTIES

The Rey Osterrieth Complex Figure can be a useful tool to visually connect a child's
day-to-day struggles with their cognitive profile. Many clinicians shared the specific ways
they use this measure to concretely demonstrate the meaning of their findings to families.
For example: If the way children have performed on the Rey suggests frontal lobe dysfunction, I ask parents to take their finger and trace how they would go about it.

o *"So you see the structure. You see this rectangle with bisecting lines. Here is what
Jane has done ... " ("Oh my God! This is exactly Jane! 'She is so disorganized.")*

—Brenda Spiegler, Ph.D.

o *(Having pulled out a copy of the figure): "Do you see this pattern—this is what he
was supposed to draw. Look how he drew all these little pieces but they're not sticking together. The same thing is happening in his reading. He is able to read phrases
or word but doesn't have a constant or a thing to hold it together. Or you notice
that he can do the problems with you in homework, but not the next day. That's
because he can do the rote thing, but he doesn't have a concept to hold it together.
So the next day, he doesn't know how to approach those same problems."*

—Deborah Waber, Ph.D.

1776 Metaphor for memory encoding

I like to use the child's performance on the Rey-Osterrieth Figure to explain how his
disorganization impacts his learning.

o *"I want to show you a perfect example of how Johnny's disorganization is probably
playing out on a day-to-day basis. I asked him to copy this picture. Now, granted,
this is a complicated picture—I would even ask you to draw it if I were testing you"*
(this often helps deflate a parent's instinct to suggest that the problems I'm sharing are just because the task is "too hard"). *"If you look at Johnny's copy, you can
see that his picture looks relatively close to the original. But, if you look at how he
drew it, we can see something else.*

*I changed pencils as he drew the picture so that I could sit here now and tell you
how he copied it. You see how he drew this part and then this part ... there seems
to be little rhyme or reason as to why he went from piece to piece. Now, after he
finished copying the design, I asked him to draw everything he could remember—
without providing any warning that I would do so (I know, it's a 'mean test,' isn't*

it?). Look how much he forgot! Now, in Johnny's case his poor performance isn't really about memory. He forgot so many details because he approached this task by trying to put together a bunch of meaningless, random details. So, when he had to remember it, it was just too much for him. It's kind of like—if I were to ask you to remember the numbers 1-7- 7- 6, if you rehearsed them, and if I don't distract you too much, you could remember them. But, if you figure out those numbers are actually 1776—if you clump them into a meaningfully organized concept—you could come back next year and say—'hey doc, 1776!'"

—*Kira Armstrong, Ph.D.*

USING LABELS

To label or not to label? For years, concern that diagnostic labels would result in lowered expectations from parents and teachers, and poor self-esteem for children, led to an avoidance of specifically naming learning disabilities. There is a generation of adults who seek neuropsychological assessment for persistent learning difficulties, who as a result, never clearly understood they had dyslexia. The pendulum has swung, and special education regulations in many states now compel school teams to be specific in naming "the problem," in order to ensure that targeted, appropriate interventions are offered. Both approaches have empowerment of students at their core, and both may have unintended disempowering effects.

o *"I know you are worried about giving your child a label, and how that may eventually limit him, rather than help him. But, I believe that identifying your child's label is important, not only to ensure that he gets the services he needs, but to help empower him. If he knows his 'label' he will be better able to jump OVER the hurdles this diagnosis typically brings rather than stumble THROUGH them."*

—*Kira Armstrong, Ph.D.*

In the 1970s, it was believed that labels were stigmatizing. No one was told they had dyslexia. Recently, one of my patients was turned down for accommodations to take the medical boards, because his IEP (Individual Education Plan) in middle school had only listed a goal of 'getting good grades' and noted he was making progress, despite the fact that test results showed classic dyslexia. So the lack of a label then hurt him now.

o *"In the 70s, labels were felt to be stigmatizing. No one was told they had dyslexia. The fear was that if you called it dyslexia, you might lose motivation to get better, or your teachers would lose motivation to teach you, or your friends would make fun of you. But now the tide has turned. It turns out that not giving something a label led to a lot of confusion. If you don't know what it is, how can you fix it or compensate? So, looking at these test results from when you were a kid, it's clear you had dyslexia back then. And you still have it."*

—*Robb Mapou, Ph.D.*

o *"Really, when you have a name for something, it's affirming. Now we can say, 'this is the reason,' rather than keeping it in a gray area, where people just throw their hands up and say, 'we don't know what's going on, there's nothing we can do.'"*

—*John J. Randolph, Ph.D.*

Providing the correct label can be therapeutic

o *"Your child is already creating his own label. For example, he may complain, 'I'm dumb.' Let's give him the right one."*

—*Kira Armstrong, Ph.D.*

WILL MY CHILD BE ABLE TO GO TO COLLEGE?

Many feedback sessions include questions from parents about whether their child will be able to attend college, or whether they will be able to attend a top tier college. Sometimes there are unrealistic expectations about their abilities. Answering these questions can be a difficult balancing act between preserving hope and creating realistic expectations.

Some patient's cognitive limitations render college an unrealistic goal. The conversation can be shifted to their ultimate goal following college. If the student wants to be in health care, or be a veterinarian or a pilot, the conversation can be turned to discussion of transition planning, sheltered workshops, etc., in that field.

o *"What do you want to do after college"? (e.g., veterinarian) Great goal! Okay, you really like working with animals—how can we get you working with animals?"*

—*Christopher J. Nicholls, Ph.D.*

Some clinicians argue, "What right do we have to say medical school is not for you?" But it's heartbreaking to see students who work so hard to get through medical school. Now they are faced with the many steps involved in managed care—and they just can't do it. It helps to walk them through what their life might look like.

o *"You could try it. But you won't have time for a life. Children? You can give up children. That's fine. Maybe don't get married. Have a housekeeper, you could do that. That's possible. You could live across the street from the hospital. Is that what you want though?"*

—*Cheryl Weinstein, Ph.D.*

ACCOMMODATIONS

"I don't want to be one of those 'sped' kids." This concern, often voiced by adolescents, is unfortunately, often reality-based. Children who require special education services are often targeted for teasing by peers. Parents understand this, and may seek to protect their child by avoiding special education services. At times, this desire to protect their children from the stigma of receiving services leads to resistance to accepting the diagnosis in the first place. Consequently, sometimes we must address both issues in order to get the child the services he or she needs.

School accommodations and stigma

o *"On one hand you can feel like it's treating you like you're different. On the other hand, this is giving you tools to succeed. Everyone needs something different. You may feel like everyone is getting the same thing—but if you talk with your friends, you will find that everyone is getting slightly different things to help them succeed."*

—Keith Owen Yeates, Ph.D.

o *"There might be a stigma associated with a learning disability diagnosis, but there's also a stigma associated with struggling in your classes."*

—Michael Santa Maria, Ph.D.

The advantages of an iep

o *"One year of a good school program is worth three years of psychotherapy."*
—Deborah Waber, Ph.D., quoting William Mitchell, Ed.D.

o *"Many kids get their self-esteem by being the first one finished. I hate it when teachers say, 'he's always the last one done, and we let him sit in the back and finish the test.' How do you think this makes him feel? He should be able to circle his name, and then be able to finish it at the next break. Because we want that to change, and we want him to know he has the time."*

—Steven Guy, Ph.D.

Driving a ferrari metaphor for the advantages of an IEP

With high-intellect children, it's helpful to use a high-performance car metaphor. This highlights to the child how they go off track, and how accommodations and extra help at school can keep the car driving at top performance.

o *"What do you know about Ferraris? They are fast, but really hard to drive. The question is, what does the driver need to know to drive that car well? ... Did you not plan properly? Did that send you into a ditch? Let's think about what else you need to know in order to drive it well."*

—Janine Stasior, Ph.D.

Technological accommodations

For very disabled children, goals that families have for their children (e.g., "we want Johnny to learn how to read") may be unrealistic. We can help parents understand this and still have hope for their child's future.

> o *"Life has become more accommodating. There's never been a better time to have an intellectual disability. That sounds funny, doesn't it? Technology is no longer an intervention—it's universally available and normalized. Therefore it seems easier for families to let go of some unrealistic goals, like reading. Let me clarify that I support literacy(!), but it has never been easier for kids who cannot read to access written language. They can access stories and information—in an accommodated way—that's no longer an accommodation. A lot of people enjoy listening to books on Audible.com or on a Kindle, and when you do it you don't look any different than anyone else. Kids who can't read can still access email, websites, literature— because you can access it without reading it"* … (Parent: "So … reading is not so essential?"). *"You're saying you want him to read, but really it sounds like you want him to have access to written language."*
>
> —*Andrew Zabel, Ph.D.*

Tutoring your own child

Some parents want to become their child's tutor. It's helpful to coach parents to take a supportive role while letting others teach. Sometimes, parents raise the idea of becoming OG certified themselves.

> o *"Please, go learn OG—we need more people to do this! But tutor someone else's kid. Your role is to be a self-esteem booster. Your job is to teach your child the joy of reading—but don't be their tutor. It will ruin your relationship."*
>
> —*Steven Guy, Ph.D.*

Homeschooling

Families homeschool their children for many reasons. Sometimes the decision is driven by religion, other times by philosophy, poor local schools, or a host of other issues that may be in play. Many times, families with multiple children will compare their child's progress to that of their siblings. Usually by the time parents get to a neuropsychologist, they are concluding that homeschooling is not working.

> o *"Let's talk about what will help your child reach her potential. I know you are using a good home school curriculum, but children with special learning needs require more specific interventions. For the learning problems that Sarah has, I have concerns that you don't have the skill set to teach her and that your curriculum will not be able to support your work with her. Kids without learning problems will learn with traditional methods, but even at traditional schools you*

need teachers with special qualifications to teach children with learning disabilities." (Sometimes I might make a comment to parents about how even though I'm trained to work with kids, I wouldn't know how to teach a child with dyslexia how to read. I say this in the vein of "Heck, I wouldn't know what to do either!" as a way to emphasize that educating children is hard and really requires specialized training).

o *[In another example, I saw a mother who had eight kids under the age of 12. The curriculum she used was computer-based. The kids had to sit at the computer and go through their module with little support. She brought in her fifth child, with significant ADHD. There was no way could this boy could initiate a module and sit through it independently]. "This self-directed learning might have worked for your other kids, but it will likely not work for Johnny because of his problems with attention. If you want to use this system, you will have to structure it so it will work for him. For example, take time out to sit down with him, and stay with him through the end of each module." (This shifts the conversation away from a philosophical discussion of homeschooling, towards a, "Do you have the time and resources to educate him in the way he needs" discussion.)*

—Jennifer Janusz, Psy.D.

COLLEGES HAVE ACCOMMODATIONS, TOO

Many families are concerned that by allowing their child accommodations in elementary or high school, they will be hobbled when they get to college. Notes, extended time, books on tape can be seen as "crutches" that will mask their problems and land them in a college program they will not be prepared for.

o *"Every college in the country has a Center for Students with Learning Disabilities. Harvard does, MIT does, so does the local community college. They all do, because it's widely understood that students with learning disabilities have a lot to offer, and programs aren't going to deny them access and benefit from their brilliance, just because they have a disability. All of the accommodations I am recommending—we can get these for Sally in whatever college program she enters. And then once she graduates from college and hits the real world—well, I guarantee you she won't choose a career that involves her sitting in lectures taking notes and memorizing information for 10 hours a day."*

—Karen Postal, Ph.D.

Transitioning students to college accommodations

I often use this metaphor when talking to teenagers about using compensatory tools to help them as they begin their transition out of high school and on to college or whatever next steps they choose to make.

○ *"Right now your mother or your parents have basically been your coach. They have advocated for you, and they have set up a team to help you get through school and to do what you need to do. What you need to do, as you're getting older and going to college" (and whatever), "you need to become your own coach, and you need to set up your own team so you can be a winner and achieve whatever you want to achieve out of life. We all have to do that. You're not unique in this way."*

—*John Beetar, Ph.D.*

When a college student doesn't want accommodations

○ *"Just don't call your mom and dad after the first month of college and say 'Mom! Dad! College is great, I have all this free time!'" (Inoculate against the idea that no one will be managing their time.) "Unlike high school, you won't always be in the same building, and you have to organize your time. That's fine, if you want to go it alone. But if you flunk out of school, and you don't do well, then your parents have the right to say, 'We won't pay for this school. You can go to a community college.'"*

—*Robb Mapou, Ph.D.*

Families shopping for accommodations

Some families come in for neuropsychological assessment specifically to obtain accommodations for their child who is about to take the Scholastic Aptitude Test (SAT) or is entering college. Often, it is entirely appropriate to seek support given their circumstances. At other times, it appears to be a search for "an edge" rather than to support significant disability. It's helpful to set up the proper expectations when they come in.

○ *"You know, you have to be disabled in relation to other people to get accommodations. The fact that Mary has not had accommodations this far will cause the college to look very skeptically at a request for accommodations. For that reason, it is probably unlikely. Fifteen years ago, schools were much more likely to say, 'She has a mild learning disability, so we'll give her accommodations.' It's not like that any more. If you are coming in for the first time at 16 or 17, let's not think just about accommodations, let's think about what else we can do to help this kid—like study strategies."*

—*Robb Mapou, Ph.D.*

When patients don't qualify for college accommodations

Medical school students and other graduate students who have had accommodations throughout school may run into a situation in which updated testing no longer provides a strong enough rationale for accommodations, or where there is a different set of rules for obtaining them.

o *"It's okay that there are new rules. You can't work with extended time. You need to learn to be more efficient. You have to have a life. Change may be necessary—and it's okay."*

—*Cheryl Weinstein, Ph.D.*

SECURING SPECIAL EDUCATION SERVICES (IEPS)

When marathon runners reach mile 20, many supporters in the crowd shout, "Great job! You're halfway there!" Of course, marathons are 26.2 miles, and the runners have long passed the halfway point. But those last six miles can seem like 13. This is an apt analogy for securing IEP services following a feedback session. Once families understand the diagnosis and have "bought into" the rationale for accommodations and services, they still have a long way to go. Neuropsychologists' recommendations have to be secured through the IEP process. Due to budget issues, IEP teams may feel pressure to keep children off the IEP rolls or to minimize services. Therefore, even when schools have the child's best interests at heart, securing necessary services can still become a protracted battle.

Securing an appropriate IEP almost always involves a negotiating process. The process might be complicated by mismatches between the family's expectations about what special education can accomplish and the reality of the severity of their child's disability. As the child progresses through school, many families will also struggle with whether to allow their educational team to shift to a focus on functional skills for their child, because they are worried that the team will expect less of their child—and therefore will provide fewer services. Helping parents develop realistic expectations and educating them about the special education process can therefore be critical components of a pediatric feedback session.

o *"We have a solid road map here for the services Andrew needs. Now the trick is to get those services through an IEP meeting. Call the school and let them know you had an independent neuropsychological evaluation and are requesting an eligibility meeting. Tell them you are dropping off a letter to officially make the request. A letter triggers a legal process where the school will need to convene a team within a specified number of days. A phone call doesn't trigger that process. Writing that letter also communicates to them that you are sophisticated about this process, and not easily brushed off.*

Many families like me to go with them to the IEP meeting, and I am happy to do so for Andrew. Another option is to attend the meeting, see what they have to offer, and if you have any reservations, don't sign anything, and let them know you will think it over. You can then call me and we can discuss next steps. Those could include calling another meeting where you invite me, or hiring an advocate.

The key is to understand that this is a negotiation process. And it's often a long and frustrating process. I want to be a resource to you all. You can call any time you have questions, and you can also give permission for me to speak with any team member who has further questions."

—*Karen Postal, Ph.D.*

The squeaky wheel metaphor for securing ieps

o *"Being a special education director is the worst job in the world. They have so much financial pressure. The law requires that children who need services get those services, but this is an 'unfunded mandate' and there are often not enough resources to go around. So it may be frustrating, but if you are persistent and strategic, in most cases you can secure those resources for your child.*

By the way, it's not fair that the 'squeaky parents' get the best services for their children, but it's true. You are much more likely to get good services now, because you are informed and motivated, and you have an independent evaluation in hand. It's not right that kids without parents like you may not get the services they need, so I encourage you all to also get involved with the local SPED PAC (Special Education Parent Committee) or" (fill in the blank for the learning disability association) *"so that you can help to change that unfair system. But in the meantime, if anyone's child will get appropriate services, it's going to be yours."*

—*Karen Postal, Ph.D.*

Educating parents to be consumers of reading services

It's important to educate families to be consumers of reading services. Even special education staff with master's degrees in reading might not be trained to administer scientifically based reading programs like Wilson or Orton-Gillingham.

o *"Here's what you have to find out. Who's working with your child—and at what intensity? This is where my expertise leaves off. I know what to recommend, because I know what the research says. There are lots of different programs. Wilson is the one of them that gives a nice certificate—here's something to hang on your wall. Qualifications."*

—*Bill MacAllister, Ph.D.*

Inviting an adolescent to the iep meeting

o *"I would really like you to be there. Sometimes people don't want to be there because they would feel uncomfortable. I understand that—the teachers will be talking about you. At the same time, they will be making decisions about your day. Your opinion is the most important one in this room."*

—*Steven Guy, Ph.D.*

Refocusing IEP Goals

With developmental disabilities and severe learning disabilities, the focus is often: "How do we help the child do schoolwork?" This can result in goals that are focused upon the past: "Mario was 60 percent accurate in simple addition last year, so let's build that to 70 percent accuracy this year."

o *"Let's ask a different question. Instead of helping the child 'do school,' how can the school help the child prepare to 'do life?' Why do we educate in the first place? We tend to be programmed to help accommodate, to intervene to help the child meet the demands of school. Let's look beyond school for a minute. I want you to visualize a realistic vision for Mario when he's 25. Where do you see him living, what do you see him doing? What about his relationships? What about his work? It's okay to have different perspectives. Let's say he is living in an apartment at 25—what would the barriers be? What are the safety concerns? Parents often fear the possibility of injury, poor initiation, social isolation, or possible exploitation in this 'future scenario.' I think these fears should be the targets of the IEP, particularly if the child is in a functional skills curriculum. Get the team to put their target in the future, and determine what needs to happen to get the child ready for it."*

—*Andrew Zabel, Ph.D.*

Shifting IEPS toward life skills

o *Parents are often scared that the school will lower their expectations for a child if he or she moves to a functional skills curriculum. Actually, this should be a conversation about raising expectations—that Mario will live as independently as possible. These are greater expectations, with a higher level of necessary service intensity. With this shift, we are (hopefully) no longer focusing on handwriting and counting coins—we are now talking about learning online banking, using an electronic calendar cueing system, using text-to-speech and speech-to-text software. We are anticipating what the self-care and daily living expectations will be like ten years in the future, rather than what they are like right now.*

—*Andrew Zabel, Ph.D.*

THE COMORBIDITY OF ANXIETY DISORDERS, ADHD, AND LEARNING DISORDERS

The referral question for a learning assessment often includes, "We aren't sure whether this [presenting problem] is a reading problem or anxiety." Of course, it's often both. Cognitive strengths and weaknesses that produce differences in learning styles also can produce differences in how children regulate and express emotions. At the same time, having a learning or developmental disability is a hard road to travel and can lead to frustration in school and at home, which over time can develop into clinical depression, or anxiety. In addition, being different can result in estrangement from their peers and put a large target on children's backs for bullying. Connecting the dots between cognitive, social, and emotional processes can significantly improve parents' relationships with their children, and their ability to advocate for their children within the school system.

- ○ *"The learning disorder and anxiety are mutually exacerbating."*
  —*Deborah Waber, Ph.D., quoting William Mitchell, Ed.D.*

Anxiety, adhd, and dyslexia

- ○ *A lot of kids have dyslexia, anxiety, and ADHD all at the same time. Their dyslexia increases their anxiety. Their anxiety decreases their frustration tolerance. Their ADHD makes it harder for them to hang in there. What takes a typical child 30 minutes, takes a kid with ADHD 45 minutes, but they were 'done' in 15 minutes, leaving 50 to 60 percent of the homework undone.*
  —*Steven Guy, Ph.D.*

Anxiety's exacerbating effects on dyslexia

- ○ *"When schools say it isn't a problem because of the 'average' testing results, I will tell you it is a problem. Sally scored in the low 90s on reading. But because of her anxiety, she will functionally read worse. School programming is not always set up to address this."*
  —*Steven Guy, Ph.D.*

Language deficits and shyness

- ○ *"Tom can't process the language quickly enough, or speak quickly enough, because he has a retrieval problem. You may see him being more reticent in social situations because he really can't assert himself."*
  —*Deborah Waber, Ph.D.*

11 Autistic Spectrum Disorders

WITH LAYERS OF social, cognitive, emotional, and educational issues, feedback with parents who have children on the autistic spectrum can be daunting. "Where to begin" is often determined by the patient's developmental stage. Is this a first diagnosis, or has the patient been involved in years of intervention? Some parents have long suspected an autism diagnosis, while others are not ready to hear the word. Helping parents and patients accept this diagnosis often requires specific education about what an autism spectrum disorder really is, or what it means. In some cases, this will help parents implement necessary interventions even if they are not ready to accept the "label."

EXPLAINING AUTISM SPECTRUM DISORDERS AND ASSOCIATED DIFFICULTIES

o *"This profile is consistent with Asperger's syndrome" (or "is on the Autistic spectrum"). "It's another kind of learning disability. It affects social learning. And it also affects school learning. As learning becomes more contextual and nuanced, the child can miss important elements, and school is a social experience. Many people don't recognize for kids how important the social environment is."*

—*Deborah Waber, Ph.D.*

It can be very hard for teachers or extended family members to understand why a child with autism might have such an extreme reaction when a favored routine is broken. Offering an explanation may help caretakers realize that the child may not simply be spoiled or stubborn.

o *"It's like the earth is tilting on its axis. It's not how you and I feel when we are disappointed that our routine is changed. But, when John's routine is changed, it's like the whole world has shifted and there is no solid ground. In that moment, he doesn't need to hear why the routine change is 'no big deal.' His world is tilted, and he needs help finding his feet, finding solid ground. He may have something special he does, something that might help him feel the world is right again."*

—*Karen Postal, Ph.D.*

Feedback sessions are an opportunity to connect the abstract diagnosis to tender points in patients' lives where they have felt upset. At the same time, it's important to talk about the strengths people have. A good strategy is to move back and forth between reminding patients about their strengths, and their areas of difficulty. In some cases tension arises between patients who have Asperger's and their family members, because of the impact of their rigidity (e.g., when a patient might be late for things, because she was lining up her toys or dressing herself to look like a certain character). It's important to remember that families may be frustrated and also afraid of this behavior, because they sometimes worry that the rigidity or oddness may represent a mental illness, even schizophrenia. Normalizing this behavior and explaining its context is critically important.

o *"You know, your mother's been very upset with you over the years. Lately she has been concerned and disturbed that you couldn't go out of the house until you had dressed like Anime—and that you would even miss dinner or going out to a party because you weren't ready and couldn't move along. You know, I think there may be a lot of reasons for why you are so focused on Anime, but I don't think the reasons need to be thought of as anything scary. A lot of people with Asperger's develop keen interests. Right now you have an interest in Anime. Maybe this could even be considered an example of an obsessive interest. But, you are not alone in that. I think your mother has the sense that you are the only person on earth who has this intense type of interest or focus. Of course, there are many, many people who are keenly interested in Anime. Some have Asperger's, some don't—but probably a fair number of them do. It might not seem so frightening to your mother if she knew that a lot of bright, productive people, without psychiatric conditions, have such interests."*

—Linda Vincent, Psy.D.

o *Asperger's is believed to be a neurodevelopmental condition that results in impairment in social and interpersonal relations. It is often characterized by narrow and obsessive interests and a pedantic or formal communication style. Once diagnosed, many individuals with Asperger's feel that these differences make them very interesting people.*

—Linda Vincent, Psy.D.

Stereotypical behaviors in autism spectrum disorders

Parents often ask why their children engage in "flapping" or other stereotypical behaviors.

o *"We think it probably feels good. We all do things that make us feel good. Some people tap their foot, or cross their legs. When people cross their legs, they get a sense of comfort. For a child with autism, it's the same kind of thing, but far more exaggerated. A typical child might bounce on their toes when excited. Your child flaps. And without good social self-monitoring, the behavior spirals—it feels better and better … so he keeps doing it."*

—Rebecca Wilson, Psy.D.

Sensory sensitivities in autism spectrum disorders

o *"There's a whole system in our body that tells us where we are in space—it's called proprioception. Even when you close your eyes, this system gives you information about how your body is oriented. You are sitting in a chair. Now, at the next level of awareness, you also can feel that you have clothes on, or sense the lighting in the room. Until I bring it up, you probably aren't aware of the feeling of your shoes on your feet, or your shirt on your arms. But some kids, with a difference in how this system is developing, may be super-aware of all of these things, all the time. They may become overwhelmed by all this input—the feel of their shoes, clothes, lighting, the chair they are sitting on. And it may be hard to focus on anything else."*

—*Rebecca Wilson, Psy.D.*

SHARING AN AUTISM DIAGNOSIS WITH PARENTS

Introducing an autism diagnosis can be a delicate task that needs to be handled with tact and a well thought-out approach. Many clinicians handle this presentation in different ways, depending on the cues the family provides regarding their readiness for this label. For example, Rebecca Wilson, Psy.D., begins the dialogue with a clear statement and then allows the process to unfold:

- o *"So, I do think your child meets criteria for autism." After I have said those words, I literally put my notebook down, and say, "I'm going to stop there for a minute." This is a concrete way of signaling, "Okay, we are now going to put the data aside." If physicians or interns are in the room with me for the feedback session, they know not to fill in that space.*

Sharing an autism diagnosis—the label is a tool to access resources

- o *"Jon meets criteria for autism.... But, It doesn't matter what we call this, it matters what we do about it ... we need to get John social pragmatics training ... " etc.*

—*Gerry Taylor, Ph.D.*

Sharing an autism diagnosis when parents are not ready to accept it

When parents are vehemently certain their child does not have autism, telling them that you see the diagnosis as autism is a tricky, difficult conversation to have. Many clinicians feel that one HAS to tell them the diagnosis even if it's clear that the parent won't accept it, even if one knows they won't come back; but I disagree.

Sometimes it is easier to say that autism is really a description of behavior, it doesn't necessarily involve mental retardation, and kids can have good outcomes. So often parents' opposition to the label turns out to be something fairly simple, or they initially sound like their defenses are three feet thick, but when we just knock on the door a little, they say, "Well, maybe you are right," and it turns out their defenses are not what they appeared to be. But if I put one foot down that road and hear the iron gate clang shut—"NO, my child does not have autism," then I just back off. I'll talk about autism, but I don't use the word. Sooner or later they will come around, but if they are telling you they aren't ready to hear it, they won't—as long as you can get them what they need without that immediate "buy-in."

○ *"You feel pretty sure you child does not have autism. Why do you think that is? What do you think autism is that doesn't describe your child? Autism is really a description of behavior; it doesn't necessarily involve mental retardation, kids can have good outcomes … and it's very important for you to know that this diagnosis can get your child very good service.*

You know your child is only two" (or three or whatever), "so we don't need to agree about diagnoses right now, but we need to worry about what are John's strengths, his weaknesses, and what he needs now."

—Deborah Fein, Ph.D.

Sometimes when the parents aren't ready to accept the diagnosis, they can accept that the report will say "Autism" or imply it in order to get the child services. You have to make an alliance with the parents and make sure they know you understand how they feel. You respect their feelings. You can let them know that you respect their opinions, but if you say this in the report, you can get the child service he needs. Then I'll write in the report that these are the criteria he meets (e.g., difficulty with eye contact, peer relationships, etc.)

○ *"Between us, we can decide to wait to see how he looks in six months or a year to decide if this is autism, but if I say in the report that the child meets criteria set up by the DSM for autism, if I say that in the report, that will get you the services you need. And the diagnosis can always be changed later."*

—Deborah Fein, Ph.D.

Sharing an autism diagnosis—it is not your fault

A generation ago, parents were told that their "cold parenting style" was the cause of their child's autism. Some parents may have heard something like this along the way, and therefore it is key to reassure them, early on, that this is not the case.

○ *"For reasons that we really don't understand, the literature is really pointing toward genetics. Some children are born with difficulties relating to others, in learning how to regulate themselves, in acquiring normal cognition. We really don't understand why, but we do know that you didn't do anything wrong and aren't to be blamed."*

—Joel Morgan, Ph.D.

DISCUSSING LONG-TERM EXPECTATIONS AND PROGNOSIS

Most parents want to know about prognosis, and many of them are too scared to ask. For some of them it's a new diagnosis; they are overwhelmed, they don't want to think about when the kid is 21 if the kid is two. They want to know what they have to do right now, or what they have to do for the next year or two. So, I won't really talk about long-term prognosis. But, depending on the cuing I am getting—if they are really struggling with, "Will my kid ever get married or go to college?" I will at least broach it.

If the child is over age seven, and has been in a good program for two years, you have some information about long-term prognosis. But if the child is younger and hasn't had enough treatment, there is not enough information to make this prognosis, and this needs to be explained to parents.

o *"You know, he's really still young, but do you want to talk about what his life will be like in the long term? Is that on your mind? There's a huge range of outcomes for children with autism. Some of them are basically indistinguishable from other adults or adolescents. Some of them have severe challenges and handicaps that they will have to deal with for the rest of their lives. That's the two ends of the continuum. So, children can range from a very limited outcome to an excellent outcome.*

Your child is unfortunately too young" (or *"you haven't done treatment long enough")* "[for us] to really know which way he is heading. So what you have to accept right now (and this is really difficult, I know) is that there is this large range of outcome and you're going to live with that uncertainty for the next few years. Now is the time to focus on the immediate future, like the next year, and give your child whatever you possibly can so that he will fulfill his potential. If you ask me two years from now, I may be able to give you more direction about where he is heading." (That usually gives them some closure even if I'm telling them there's no closure yet.)*

—Deborah Fein, Ph.D.

For children who have autistic disorders, their long-term prognosis is often predicted more by their intellectual abilities than by their autism. If parents ask whether their child will get married when the prognostic signs suggest otherwise, it's important to address the question directly.

o *(For a child with significant intellectual handicaps or severe autism): "It is very unlikely that he will be able to get married, but he will be able to have relationships with peers and maybe even have sex if interested. But he will always need someone to look after him."*

—Deborah Fein, Ph.D.

Moving back to the farm metaphor to reassure parents of children with autism spectrum diagnoses

This is a wonderful way of normalizing a lack of social skills and reassuring parents that this challenge does not have to define their child.

o *"For hundreds of years, we were a farming society. And we may have had a lot of kids with autism, but they were farming. There was no requirement for great social skills out on the farm. And then for the past 200 years, with the Industrial Revolution, we have had an intensely interactive society. And that's unnatural,*

*and really stressed kids with your son's issues. Now we are 'returning to the farm.'
But the 'farm' is now the computer. We are moving back toward less human inter-
activity, which gives your child an opportunity. He can have an entire social life
without any face-to-face human interactions."*

—Tom Boll, Ph.D.

RECOMMENDATIONS AND INTERVENTIONS

Understanding the different needs and interests of children with autism spectrum disorders

In a typical case of moderate Asperger's, the teenage boy or young adult is fine with less interaction. Particularly for the mothers, this is important to explain. This message can be delivered in front of the teenager. Many teens are hugely relieved when this is brought out in the open: "See, Mom? I'm fine."

o *"Parents can inappropriately attribute distress where it doesn't exist. You know he
is not nearly as upset as you are. That's part of the syndrome. You want him to be
out and engaged with other people. You go on vacation and he stays in the room
the whole time. And you think he's not enjoying himself because he is not doing
what the other kids are doing. But he's fine. Even though you are in Hawaii and
he is by himself or in the hotel room the whole time, he's not unhappy. You are
assuming that he experiences his emotions and thinks in the same way as most
people, but he doesn't. It is so unique. It's so hard to understand how he feels,
because he doesn't feel like you and I do about things. He just doesn't have that
expressiveness. Now, he does experience fear and anxiety and worry—that's often
more prevalent in Asperger's and it's important to be sensitive to those emotions.
But in a weird way, you can't really put yourself in his shoes and assume that he
is feeling what you are feeling. It's a sad thing that he doesn't feel like other people
do, but in a way it's also a good thing because he is not nearly as distressed as you
think he is. And that can take the pressure off of your having to worry so much
about him, at least on that issue."*

—Jim Irby, Ph.D.

When treating the child at the expense of the family

Families may throw all their resources behind the child in their family who is severely impaired, severely retarded, or severely autistic. It's good for the child, but sometimes it's not going to make a tremendous difference for him, and it's often at the cost of the marriage or the siblings. For example, when I was working with one family, everything revolved around the autistic child—the siblings were not getting play dates, they were expected to parent the affected child and give up some of their normal childhood activities and relationships. In this example, everyone wanted to go on a trip, and they had the money to make the trip. But the affected child could not have gone. So they decided not to go. I spoke to them about trying to balance the needs of the other children.

> o *"It's going to be important for Johnny to have a family that is happy and functional and that the other kids get what they need and don't become resentful, because he will be relying on them in the long run."*
>
> —Deborah Fein, Ph.D.

When the family has an autistic child and the sibling has special, but less severe, needs, often the sibling's needs don't get met. One role of the neuropsychologist during feedback can be to broaden the discussion of needs and services to the other siblings.

> o *"Your other child has ADHD and she has some social issues, so she needs some extra help as well. I know this isn't what you came here for, but the whole family is important and we should talk about her, too."*
>
> —Deborah Fein, Ph.D.

ALTERNATIVE TREATMENTS

Parents whose children have special needs are often willing to consider any intervention possible to help their child. Many brokers of alternative therapies or "treatments" take advantage of this desire and offer families promises of "cures," often at exorbitant costs and at times, even potential risks for the child. It can be important to help parents select the best treatment options, while simultaneously balancing their needs for hope.

Alternative treatments—understanding the parents' need to leave no stone unturned

> o *Sometimes it's important for us to remember that for their own future, sometimes parents have to feel like they did everything possible, so they're not tortured by the fact that they had not done x, y, or z—that he might have been better.*
>
> —Deborah Fein, Ph.D.

When discussing fringe interventions for autism (e.g., chelation, diets, horseback riding), I want to communicate that I understand their desperation.

> o *"You know, I'm sure if it were my kid I would be trying everything, too."*
>
> —Deborah Fein, Ph.D.

When parents are committed to alternative medical interventions

I often hear about this when parents are talking about quack treatments. The problem is that a lot of these are dispersed by doctors, and I'm not an M.D. I'm very scrupulous about providing medical advice. If I am asked by a parent about medication, my immediate answer is, "I'm not an M.D."

- o *"I'm not an M.D., so I'm not going to tell you to do it or not do it. Have you spoken to your pediatrician about it?" (They usually say yes.) "I can't give you medical advice, but I can tell you that this particular treatment—from everything I've read about it, there's not a lot of evidence to support it. The most important thing is to do no harm, so I really think you should talk to your pediatrician about whether there could be anything harmful about it. Aside from medical harm, another kind of harm is that you take time, money, and resources away from things that you know can be effective to[spend on] things that are less supported by evidence. So, if you're giving your child this intervention that you feel may be important, don't stop the behavioral intervention."*

—*Deborah Fein, Ph.D.*

Gluten/casein-free diet

When parents tell me they have put their child on a gluten/casein-free diet, it's really difficult, because of course you want to say—stop doing this treatment that has no evidence and is socially and nutritionally restricting! Unless, of course, the child has a medically documented illness like celiac disease. I won't say this because it is a medical treatment. But I will point them to the evidence, help them set up a structured trial, and tell them not to drop the evidence-based treatment.

- o *"One possibility, and you should discuss this with the prescribing doctor, you could do a trial where you give the kid a small challenge of the ingredient (like one wheat cracker) and ask the teacher to keep track of the child's attention, behavior, eye contact, a few things. Don't tell them when you are challenging the child and when you are not. That may allow you to see what effect the diet is really having. I could help you set up a rating scale to give to the teachers to see if this is effective. But of course you need to consult the supervision doctor first."*

—*Deborah Fein, Ph.D.*

Diet treatments

This pearl is appropriate for any condition, including autism, where special diets might be entertained by parents as alternative treatments.

- o *"I take medication for my cholesterol. I didn't know at first that I can't eat grapefruit with this medication. I would never have thought about that. Whatever you do, you need to talk to your child's doctor first, making sure your child gets enough nutrients. Nutrition is complex for the developing child, and taking away major food sources could have consequences you would never have thought of."*

—*Jacobus Donders, Ph.D.*

LONG-TERM PLANNING FOR AUTISTIC CHILDREN

This topic is addressed in Chapter 10 ("Developmental Disabilities"); many of the pearls and metaphors in that chapter are applicable to this population as well.

ISSUES SPECIFIC TO ADULTS WITH AUTISTIC SPECTRUM DISORDERS

Some adults with Asperger's come into the office having already read a lot about it, and they self-identify. Diagnostic feedback for that group is relatively easy because they have made a connection between what they have been reading and their own situation. It is helpful to begin by congratulating them for being insightful and for identifying some of the issues in their lives.

> o *"One of the things that I want to tell you right from the beginning—and not have you anticipate over the hours—I am going to agree with a lot of the things that you have been thinking about yourself. And I really admire the insightfulness that you have had about realizing the basis for some of the problems in your life."*
>
> —Linda Vincent, Psy.D.

The benefits of differential diagnosis from the patient's perspective: would this diagnosis be limiting or liberating?

A diagnosis is more or less useful depending on how it leads to the next step in the patient's life. In some cases a diagnosis may be very limiting. In others it is very liberating because it allows an individual to understand some of the problems they are having in everyday life.

> o *"Asperger's exists on a spectrum. There are aspects on your testing profile and in your clinical history that are consistent with this diagnosis and some that are not. Do you think that having the diagnosis will be limiting or liberating for you? How would it be helpful for you in your everyday life?"*
>
> —Margaret O'Connor, Ph.D.

Diagnosing adults with autism spectrum diagnosis—why did it take so long?

When an adult is diagnosed with Asperger's or an autism spectrum disorder, the discussion often turns to other family members with similar characteristics—a parent, an uncle who was "eccentric." Sometimes there is a feeling of blame: "Why didn't someone pick this up before?"

> o *"Asperger's tends to run in the family. Maybe this wasn't recognized—because in your family, maybe you weren't so different from your father."*
>
> —Linda Vincent, Psy.D.

Helping spouses understand unique deficits in autism spectrum disorders

Often couples are seen together for feedback sessions. It's common for the wife to express frustration. She might feel that her husband is being intentionally difficult, not really wanting a relationship—or not putting out for a relationship. She may be hurt by all the things that are not happening—like birthdays not being recognized. When she becomes upset, she may feel that her husband does not always know how to relate to her in a helpful way. One strategy that both explains the core deficits in Asperger's syndrome and helps relieve the spouse's frustrations is to contrast the intellect with the social skills deficits; start with the strengths, then contrast those strengths with the challenges in relationship skills.

> o *"What a contrast it is. That someone who is so bright, so intelligent, could have such a hard time in the social world and with relationships. That is really confusing—not only for you—but for your family, your spouse. How odd this is, [that] a person like you who is so intelligent, wouldn't know what to do when he finds his wife crying. Sometimes what you do or say just makes it worse, even when you don't mean to do that. It's not your intention, but that can be the outcome." (At this point, try to bring in specific examples to try to bridge to the diagnosis).*
> —*Linda Vincent, Psy.D.*

Feedback can often become a couples-counseling session—in that it is a wonderful opportunity for building empathy. When one person in the couple is diagnosed with Asperger's, feedback sessions can be emotional. In my experience, usually the wife is the neurotypical—and when she begins to learn about Asperger's, the light bulb goes on. Sometimes this can be a positive realization, but other times the wife may feel a great deal of guilt by recognizing all of the misattributions she has made. Recently the wife of a man I diagnosed with Asperger's said, "Oh, damn! You are killing me, now I can't be as mad at him!"

> o *We all make up stories to explain what is not directly evident to us—we try to fill in the gaps to make sense of it all. So, we make attributions when someone has been unresponsive, or been hurtful, or said something peculiar, or done something we don't like. The story we make up about that person may not be accurate, but we are just trying to fill in the gaps, to make meaning.*
> —*Linda Vincent, Psy.D.*

12 Acquired Brain Injury: traumatic Brain Injury and Cerebrovascular Accidents

(Countinued)

APPROACHES TO FEEDBACK regarding acquired brain injuries vary, depending on patient characteristics such as lesion location, injury severity, time since injury, and the patient's developmental lifespan stage. A theme that emerged among many of the techniques was the goal of preserving hope, while clearly addressing the patient's injuries and limitations. Many of the pearls in this chapter were presented to us with an emphasis on either traumatic brain injury (TBI) or cerebrovascular accident (CVA), even when their content may be appropriately applied to both populations. We present both sets of pearls together in this chapter because of the common issues stemming from a sudden, unexpected, acquired brain injury. (Additional approaches to addressing unawareness of deficits can also be found in Chapter 6: "Dementia").

DISCUSSING PROGNOSIS AND EXPECTATIONS FOR RECOVERY

Providing feedback to families and patients who have sustained moderate or severe TBI or CVAs often involves sharing bad news. Being blunt is sometimes appropriate and even necessary, particularly when safety is an issue. At other times, especially early in the recovery course, it is not helpful to confront the families with how bad the outcome is likely to be. They typically don't want to hear it, and they may not be emotionally ready to cope with that message. A tension emerges between providing sufficient information and allowing a process of gradual discovery and acceptance. Acknowledging there is much about brain recovery we do not understand can be helpful in softening the prognosis message. Neuropsychologists can also actively invite patients and families to look at the positive changes as well as the persisting deficits.

Explaining the TBI recovery curve

o *"Let me just remind you, encourage you to understand that TBI is a lot different from something like Alzheimer's, which you might have heard about. First of all, Alzheimer's disease is an illness. And it gets worse over time. It's progressive. In your case you have a TBI. It's an accident. The worst of it is in the beginning. Over time it can get better. And that is something to hold on to. I can't guarantee; I don't know exactly how far it will go, but in general things get better over time."*
—Tony Wong, Ph.D.

o *"You will continue to improve, but it will be in smaller increments over longer periods of time. This is how much you're getting back."* (While drawing curve and plotting milestones,) *"Here you were almost dead—you were in a coma. Then you woke up—here's a big jump. Here you first started using your voice—a big jump. And here you started to walk, that's a BIG jump. Now, you see it's still going up? But it's not going up as fast as it was. Okay, see how long it took to get 10 percent back? In the beginning it only took you a week. Now, to get 10 percent more, it takes you three months.*
—Jacobus Donders, Ph.D.

Explaining recovery of awareness

o *When you first came out of the injury, you didn't even realize that you were in the hospital. When you were able to say where you were and that you had been in an accident—that's the first level of awareness. Then, being able to describe how you have been affected by the injury—like your right arm is weak, and your memory is affected. That's another level of awareness. Then there's the level of being able to appreciate how this will affect your daily life. That's one of the top levels of awareness—and of course some people don't have that even if they never had a brain injury."*

—*Jim Irby, Ph.D.*

Explaining developmental trajectory in children

o *(Drawing a graph.) "Here is mental age, and here is developmental age. All of our tests are designed so that with each increment in developmental age, there's equal increment with mental age. You get a 45-degree angle. So here is the injury—and there's now been a drop. What we're going to do over the next several years, we're going to plot his development. We're going to see if it comes back up to the line, or parallel to the line. Because in some cases it won't come all the way back. It stays down. If it doesn't come up, it may look like he's getting worse, but he's not, the test scores are just staying down, and he looks worse compared to his peers."*

—*Erin D. Bigler, Ph.D.*

Family support as a predictor of outcome after brain injury

o *There are many things about the brain that we don't understand. The ways that the brain adapts to injury—we are just beginning to understand. So it is very difficult to predict an outcome. But there are two predictors that we know about. The first is severity—that is, how long your child was in coma. The second one is the amount of family support. There's not much we can do now about the severity of the injury"* (the depth of coma or length of post traumatic amnesia). *"That's over. What we want to concentrate on is how is the quality and nature of the family support, and other resources that I can help you line up in helping Joey optimize his recovery."*

—*Paul Kaufmann, J.D., Ph.D.*

Set up an expectation for improvement

o *"What are some of the things that you are noticing are improving? What are you getting better at? What have been the positive outcomes from the accident? The good news with TBI is that there is improvement."* (For moderate to severe TBI,) *"You may not get back entirely to where you were before, but there is improvement."* (I then go into their strengths in the neuropsychological profile).

—*Robin Hanks, Ph.D.*

Why prognosis is difficult to predict

○ *"The brain and the spinal cord are the only tissues in our body that don't grow new cells as the main way to recuperate. If you break a bone, we grow new cells from our marrow, that's why the doctors can say, 'In six weeks you will be good as new!' With brains, you never hear anybody give you a straight answer like that. And that's because they really don't know. In any brain injury, some cells die, but some are just injured. The cells look like a tree. They have a cell body, and arms that look like a tree—and they connect with other cells to form neural networks. So healing will occur, but the cells that are dead stay dead. And that's why you can't get a straight answer early on because no one really know the proportions—and time will tell."*

—Barbara Schrock, Ph.D.

CREATING REALISTIC EXPECTATIONS FOR TREATMENT AND LONGER-TERM GOALS

This can be a good way to present tough prognoses without closing the door of hope. "Jack is not going to be able to go back to school," vs. "Let's see where we are in a few months." One of the narratives all patients and families have, and should have, is "We're going to beat the odds." "The doctor said I would never walk again, and I did." It's there for a good reason. That balance between being brutally frank, vs. allowing patients to discover limitations on their own, is important to honor so you can maintain your therapeutic alliance. If you lean too far in one direction, they aren't being protected. If you go too far in the other direction, they might reject what you have to say and even refuse to work with you. You don't have to give them everything at once.

○ *"Let's hope for the best and plan for the worst. Just in case—I'm not saying this will happen, but just in case—here's what we need to be ready for. I think that the most likely outcome or problem you might have to deal with is this. I'm not sure if I'm right. I may be right, I may be wrong. I hope you can prove me wrong. But I have to say, I wouldn't try to go back to school right now. That's my professional opinion. But if you are going to do it anyway, you need to be aware of these things. Here's how you are most likely to make a mistake."*

—Jim Irby, Ph.D.

Something to think about: *We don't want to leave patients hanging out to dry, and not give them difficult information that is crucial to planning and safety. At the same time, rather than clobbering them with brutal information, it's often best to let them come to their own acceptance. For this reason, I speak in terms of probability. I might qualify it and say something like "highly likely," but I avoid speaking in definitive terms: "Here's what I think is probably going to happen."*

—Jim Irby, Ph.D.

Families of TBI patients can remain in denial, even after hearing about an IQ in the 70s after a severe TBI. They may say to themselves and their child, "You're still going to be a cardiac surgeon!" There is nothing to be accomplished by taking away all their hope, but one can foreshadow—"college will be very difficult"—and then refocus on realistic current expectations.

> o *"Well, why don't we talk a little bit about how we're going to get Sarah through her junior year in high school? Look, I'm going to tell you some things you won't like to hear. And I am going to qualify them by saying I'm not God and I don't know everything and can't see into the future. But we're going to have some problems in the future. And we're going to shoot for getting her through her junior year. What I want to see in three months or six months is this—and if it looks better, great. We don't have to settle for just this or that this is the way it's going to be forever. But college—grad school is very far off. And if you ask me" (they did) "I think it's going to be very challenging. Let's focus on where we are now, which is finishing her junior year."*
>
> —Jacobus Donders, Ph.D.

Talking with Patients About Being Dependent

With severe TBI or a significantly limiting CVA it's important to get into a frank discussion of what the resource network will be. How will they engage in a lifestyle that is pretty dependent on others? This elicits various reactions. Some say, "No way, I'm not going to need that!" Clinicians at this point can explore the resistances. Others will begin to talk about spiritual resources, etc. The key thing is to make the statement, then give the patient and family time to talk. Feedback is not just about hearing the brilliant neuropsychologist. It's a chance for patients and families to talk about their plans, informed by the test findings.

> o *"So you survived. Now what's going to happen? Where are you going to get the support that you are going to need? Gee, we've got to understand that you will be dependent on others for the foreseeable future."*
>
> —Robert M. Bilder, Ph.D.

Encouraging a Step-by-Step Approach to Recovery

A step-by-step approach allows people to focus on what they are capable of doing currently, as opposed to what they cannot do.

> o *"The way you are going to get to your goal is by one-step-at-a-time action. And you have to stick with actions that you really can do now. You keep on working on the things you can do today. And keep on working on it for the rest of the week, and next week you probably are going to be able to do more. Just keep on working on it week after week. And over months, you will see improvement, and year after year you will continue to see improvement."*
>
> —Robert M. Bilder, P.D.

OFFERING HOPE

Sharing a Successful Example to Foster Hope

Sometimes sharing success stories can be helpful for families. This story is of a teenager who was so well known in the larger community that I feel comfortable sharing at this level of detail. There are two threads of the story—1) There's hope for amazing gains, way beyond what we predicted, and 2) **But** he still has deficits. Storytelling directs people back to "We don't know what the outcome will be."

o *"We're still in the short term. Recovery is a long-term process. Let me tell you about one of our former patients. This kid was a high school senior, star football player, aggressively recruited by Big Ten teams. He was entirely sober, but driving his drunk friend home quickly so he could make his curfew. The car flipped. Ironically, the intoxicated friend was not injured. The patient ended up with a Glasgow Coma Scale score of 3. One of the worst acute scans I had ever seen. Every kind of neuropathology you can think of in a several-day period. This person was in the deepest possible coma you can have without being dead. The family was going to put him in a nursing home from acute care. It seemed to be the most logical decision; this was an amazingly severe case. The kid was completely nonresponsive. No signs. As a matter of routine at the medical center, they always want a PM&R doctor to take a look at patients—even if the decision for nursing home care has been made. And this doctor, she noticed some minimal responsiveness, and decided to recommend the patient be put on a psycho-stimulant. Although he was still very impaired, he came around a lot more—enough that we were able to get 10-day trial of rehab approved. He started making very impressive gains in inpatient rehab. At first it was gradual. Then, when the medication was bumped up more, it literally woke him up. He became verbal and interactive. Then he really made tremendous gains. This was someone who had more family and social support than I had ever seen, to the point that they had to figure out visiting schedules because it was almost getting out of hand with his large extended family, church group, team, friends. The therapists were very motivated, as he was making measurable gains.*

"Now this individual was originally going to be a college athlete. That did not occur. He had physical issues. But he was able to get back to community college, a course at a time. He will be transferring to a full-blown university his senior year. We will see how that goes. He has measurable cognitive impairment. But has been able to pull a 'B' average double major in psychology and early education. He has had issues about disinhibition, impulsivity, acting out—things that are hard to differentiate at times from normal early 20s. But overall, considering that this was someone they thought was going to die, then at a nursing home at 18. . . . "

(Sometimes this story can be truncated—"Everyone thought he would be in a nursing home; now he's a senior in college.")

—*Joseph H. Ricker, Ph.D.*

When dealing with a highly educated, high-functioning patients, these stories can be very helpful. They tend to be more powerful than just study data or statistics. Some former patients will volunteer to talk to new patients, but they need to be carefully selected; the TBI patients who are so disinhibited or unaware—never ask them speak with new TBI patients!

> o *"I had a classmate in grad school. He fell on an icy sidewalk and sustained a moderate TBI with significant findings on his brain scan. He finished graduate school on time. I also had a post-doctoral fellow I worked with who had a significant brain injury due to a bicycle accident. She ended up finishing grad school. She now directs a clinical psych program."*
>
> —Joseph H. Ricker, Ph.D.

UNAWARENESS FOLLOWING ACQUIRED BRAIN INJURY

Addressing lack of insight into cognitive deficits and personality changes is an enormous challenge following traumatic brain injury and stroke. Lack of awareness of one's deficits can lead to serious safety concerns, as well as poorly thought-out decisions, such as a premature return to work, that might jeopardize future reintegration into the community. Poor awareness reduces motivation to participate in rehabilitation and can cause significant stresses within families when patients return home. (For pearls relating to driving, please refer to the chapter on dementia.)

> o *"One of the symptoms of a brain injury is that you are not aware of how severely impaired you are. You know how I told you the brain is the organ of memory? It's also the organ of awareness. All of your awareness is processed through your brain. If the part of your brain that processes awareness gets hurt—you won't be fully aware of what happened."*
>
> —Joseph H. Ricker, Ph.D.

Improving awareness during the initial post-injury months

> o *"Do you remember how you were three months ago? Can you think back on how you thought you were doing great? But now when you look back on how you were three months ago, you realize you are so much better right now than you were then. But do you remember three months ago, you thought you were fine? So let's think about that. What are you going to be saying in another three months? Do you think that you might be looking back on where you are now, and saying, 'boy, I had some problems!'—and realize that you still have problems. Because three months ago you said you were fine. And now you can look back and see that you were really having some problems. You can see it now. So, what do you think in three months … Do you think you will look back on where you are today and think you have gotten better?"*
>
> —Jim Irby, Ph.D.

Guys like them metaphor to improve awareness

It's much less threatening to talk about patients who are like your patient who have gone through the same thing than to confront the impaired awareness head-on.

o *"Now, let me tell you about my experience. I've worked with a lot of guys your age who have had these kinds of problems" (here is where you shift to talking about someone who is like them, but not them). "Now you may or may not fit this. I'm not saying you do. But let's talk about others who have had this type of injury. Here's how it goes...."*

—Jim Irby, Ph.D.

Joining with unawareness

This is usually a good way of normalizing the experience of impaired awareness. I use this statement again and again throughout the feedback, almost like a mantra: "There's nothing like a brain injury! There's no injury like it. It's not like breaking your leg."

o *"This isn't just you being oblivious.... Initially, you can't see the forest for the trees. Everyone else can notice that you're having problems with your memory. Or that your personality is different—more irritable or edgy. But a lot of people who have had a brain injury, initially they can't tell either. And I would be the same way. I even know a lot about recovering from a brain injury, but if I had one, I would be the same way. I would be thinking, 'I am ready to go back to work!' And everybody else sitting in the room would be shaking their heads—'No he's not!' Because this is how brain injuries are...."*

—Jim Irby, Ph.D.

Improving awareness by rehearsing information

Both unawareness and poor recall are barriers for TBI patients to leave a feedback session with a clear understanding of their deficits and strengths. Beginning with the patient alone in the feedback session, and then bringing family members into the session, creates an excellent opportunity to have the patient "practice the information." The idea is to have the patient tell his or her family the results of the assessment when they come into the room. This can be a powerful thing to do: Give feedback to the brain-injured patient. Then you attempt to have them explain what we have discussed with their family.

o *"I'm going to put you on the spot. Just do the best you can. I want to see how well you can tell your family what we have been talking about." (I won't let them stew in it for too long—I will jump in. People are rarely accurate). "Before I have your family come in, tell me what you are going to tell them." (That way, it gives them several opportunities to encode it, and then give it to someone else. If the patient can't, I will jump in and say, "Now here's what we found").*

Because they have now said it multiple times, they might remember it and even own it.

—*Jim Irby, Ph.D.*

Use of frontal systems behavior scale to improve awareness

A helpful way to find solid ground in discussing deficits is to have families and patients fill out the Frontal Systems Behavior Scale (FrSBe) (Grace & Malloy, 2001). The result graphs on the FrSBe can be presented to the family members to compare results. The point is to discuss people's perspective on the shared problem.

    o *"People are seeing things differently. Sue" (wife), "you are showing a lot of concern about what is happening. Tom" (patient) "is not admitting much is happening. And kids, you are showing something in-between" (then wait to see what everyone says—in most cases, people in the session agree there is some midrange appropriate for what's happening).*

—*David E. Tupper, Ph.D.*

ADDRESSING RESISTANCE WITH UNAWARE PATIENTS

    o *If someone is resistant to feedback, I'll honor that by saying: "Now you don't have to agree with me, it's my opinion. But I will say I've been doing this for a while, and I know a lot about it. You can take it or leave it. My goal is to give you my honest professional opinion and the best information I can, based on my experience. You can do with it what you want. My goal is to help you."*

—*Jim Irby, Ph.D.*

RETURN TO WORK OR SCHOOL

Ironically, while many mild traumatic brain injury patients are very concerned that they are unable to perform their typical work, severely brain-injured and stroke patients are often *overly* confident about their ability to return to work. Part of this is due to unawareness of deficits, and part is likely associated with their desire to return to normal life as soon as possible. Premorbidly very high-functioning individuals, such as attorneys, upper-level executives, or doctors, are often mistakenly convinced that after only a few weeks of rest, they can go back to work. (These patients may be working on their laptop in the rehab hospital.)

One role of the neuropsychologist is to help protect severely injured patients from the failure and discouragement that would result from returning to work or school prematurely. In addition to having an impact on their financial viability and educational progress, such failure can (depending on the nature of the patient's injury) unnecessarily trigger a loss of confidence that interferes with their later integration into the community. Messages often involve graded return to activities associated with work or school, and then graded return to work or school sites. Delivery is key, as patients might dismiss clinicians' messages if there is too large of a disconnect between their own confidence and the caution being recommended by the clinician.

Helping patients recognize when it is too early to return to work

o *"I know you feel ready to go back to work. And we want you to go back to work. I want you to get back as soon as you can. These tests will tell us where your thinking skills are, because, if there is a problem, you need to know. This is for you—you might not know about these problems. Now I've seen guys after an injury, and they don't quite realize how impaired they are within the first few months of their injury. They think they are fine. I've seen guys go back to work too soon. They end up having problems on the job, and everyone thinks it's because of the injury. And it is. But the problem is that they weren't fully recovered and they went back too soon and they blew their job.*

Now, you are still getting better. You will be getting a lot better in the next few months. If you go back before you're ready, you could blow your job too, if you go back too soon. Everybody at work will think this is where you are permanently. But it's not how you are permanently. This is where you are now. In six months you will be a lot better. And that's when it might be best to go back—because your thinking will be so much clearer. We want you to go back as soon as you are ready. I know it's frustrating being held back, but it would be more frustrating for you to go back before you're ready and lose your job and have everybody thinking that you've got permanent problems from your brain injury when you still have a lot of improvement to go."

—Jim Irby, Ph.D.

o *"What if you go back and you miss something, and you lose your case"* (in this example, the patient was an attorney)—*"how will you feel? How are the partners going to feel? I don't get paid any more for keeping you out of work than if I said, 'Okay, go back tomorrow.' I have no financial stake. I don't want you to do something to mess up your job or mess up your recovery. Going back to work too soon might even slow things down for you."*

—Joseph H. Ricker, Ph.D.

Part of the issue in helping patients with the return to work decision is understanding what work meant to them. Was work something that was a big part of their identity, or just something they hated and wanted to get through? Another critical factor is what resources they have. Do they have access to short-term disability support? Are they financially able to not return? And, what type of support exists at work? Some employers will say you can only come back full-time. Other employers say, "We'll make it work and bend over backwards." It is important for the neuropsychologist to try to learn as much as possible about these variables prior to deciding how to talk with the person about returning to work; it's also important to find out what the realistic limitations are. Is the patient the primary breadwinner? Is her husband already on disability?

o *"I know you want to go back to work and in fact in the long run I think that will be very therapeutic for you. You're not the type of person who can just sit on the couch. You'll drive yourself and your wife nuts. I also know that you want to do a good job. And I don't want to set you up for a situation in which you will screw it up. Right now I don't want you to go into a situation where you might bite off more that you can chew."* (I will have found out in the interview whether there is an option of returning with limited hours, as well as specifics of the job—how much is routine, can he do it in his sleep? How much is troubleshooting?)

—*Jacobus Donders, Ph.D.*

Broken leg metaphor for return to work

Following a TBI or stroke, the injury can be "invisible." Most people have known someone with a broken limb. This metaphor is helpful regarding pacing.

o *"You wouldn't just run around the track right after you broke your leg. You'd wear a cast for a while; then you'd get it off and probably limp for a while; and it would take you a while to work back up to running. The same thing is true for your brain. You need to give yourself time to recover before you do the equivalent of running on it"* (like going to college!).

—*Hillary Shurtleff, Ph.D.*

Spare tire metaphor for return to work

o *"You know what? I drive home from work every day, and I have a spare tire in the back of my car. I hope I never have to use it, but if I have a flat, I will be very glad I have that spare tire in the back of my care. Let's talk about 'Plan B.' Let's assume you're right. Let's assume there's nothing wrong with you. Let's assume all the doctors are stupid. But that's like assuming that you will never use that spare tire. Let's bring that spare tire along, as a safety measure, something to fall back on, just in case something does go wrong. So before you return to work or school, let's talk about some Plan B strategies."*

—*Jacobus Donders, Ph.D.*

Avoiding unnecessary discouragement when discussing return to school

Due to the risk of post-TBI depression, I want to be very careful not to say anything that will add one more thing to the patient's list of stressors.

o *("Doc, can I go back to school next semester?")* *"We're going to have to wait and see. I've been wrong, before. There are some people that I thought couldn't and they did great."*

—*Joseph H. Ricker, Ph.D.*

Asking patients to be the expert in return to work decisions

o *"If you were me, looking at these scores, what would you say about whether you could go back to work?" (Most patients say, "Yeah, I guess I would say you can't go.")*
—Dominic Carone, Ph.D.

Presenting return to work as a stepwise process

o *"We are all rooting for you to get back to work in the same way you used to. But let's think about what's the next practical step that you can take—given that you can't walk yet" (you can't move your left arm/can't talk) "You will need to complement this with all your rehab activities. Let's look at how we can get you there. What's the most sensible plan, that takes you there, one step at a time?"*
—Robert M. Bilder, Ph.D.

This works best when the patient is more senior at work and can delegate.

o *"You say you are going to go back in two weeks. Why don't we contract for six weeks. Then come back for more testing. Is there a junior partner that can take care of this? Can you delegate?"*
—Joseph H. Ricker, Ph.D.

"Flip chart of self-assessment" technique for return to work

Yehuda Ben-Yishay, Ph.D., used this approach in his small group exercises When discussing vocational readiness. This is one way to help patients think through the problem of when they are ready to go back to work. I purposely put stamina on the chart, because people generally don't think about stamina. If they are unaware, and rate themselves a 6 in terms of stamina or memory, and the staff knows they are a 2, then this discrepancy is shared with the rehab team. Team members can thereafter make sure they are giving feedback about stamina in their various areas. They can offer reality checks after asking, "how do you think you did?"

o *"Let's go through all the constructs—motor function, fine–gross, info processing, language, then social interaction, getting along with peers, authority figures, self control, self awareness." (Have a poster/ flip chart.) "Let's do it together, and define each of these constructs" (point to "Gross Motor Coordination"). "Now you are going to rate yourself on gross motor—whole body movements. Lifting, walking, carrying, balancing. Okay, if a hundred people walked in this room right now, at your age, gender, education level—where would you fall?" (When they are done with their profile, take "Jobs" and do the same thing.) "How good does a person have to be in gross motor to do that job? For example, I have a bad back, I rate myself low on gross motor. Here, this job of warehouse man: I can't do this job. I'm smart enough, but you have to be at least a 5 and I am a 3 on gross motor."*
—Barbara Schrock, Ph.D.

Pole vaulting metaphor for return to work and school

Families and patients with unrealistic expectations regarding returning to school or work may respond to sports metaphors, particularly if their child was an athlete. In this case the metaphor is of pole-vaulting, because the patient to whom it was directed was a very successful state champion pole-vaulter prior to her TBI. Other sports could be substituted. Crafting the metaphor to fit the person is powerful.

> o *"Right now you're walking with a walker. If you want to go back to pole vaulting, let's first start with walking without a walker. It's kind of like school. Let's first focus on getting through high school, rather than looking at college right now."*
> —*Jacobus Donders, Ph.D.*

HOW TO ENCOURAGE COMPENSATORY STRATEGIES AND ACTIVE REHABILITATION

Addressing compensatory strategies for cognitive deficits is an important part of feedback sessions for most neurocognitive conditions. Some of the strategies are designed to improve function, and others to inoculate against frustration. The following are particularly helpful in the context of acquired brain injury.

Juggling metaphor for compensatory techniques

> o *"What does your frontal lobe do? It juggles. Where the kids are, what you need to do at work, when your dentist appointment is.... The TBI affected how well your frontal lobe can juggle. So what we need to do is teach you some new juggling techniques"* (like block scheduling) *"and we also need to reduce the number of balls you need to keep in the air."*
> —*Susan McPherson, Ph.D.*

Plan on an extra 10 minutes – a compensatory technique

> o *"You are going to be a little rusty. It took you an hour to read a chapter before. Just plan on it taking you an hour and 10 minutes. Plan on it. Take a break. You were the kind of guy who could just look at a chapter; kind of glance over it. Now you have to work harder for it. Just plan on it."*
> —*Jacobus Donders, Ph.D.*

Encouraging self assessment to facilitate compensatory strategies

This helps patients become active participants in the rehab process. Good rehabilitation involves recruiting patients as good self-assessors.

> o *"You can't make a weakness better unless you know it's there, and you can't use your strengths unless you know what they are. Good rehab is about being a good*

self-assessor. Being able to assess yourself on a daily basis—because people are in and out of our system so quickly, that when the decisions need to be made" (return to work, return to school, return to driving)—"most of the time, they are out of our hands. So we need to give you a framework—a set of tools—'how do I know when I'm ready?'"

—Barbara Schrock, Ph.D.

With CVA and TBI, residual symptoms are often "invisible" to others (and at times to patients).

o *"You know, you are going to fool people: you can walk and talk. People want you to be well. So on the surface, it will seem that there are no symptoms from the stroke. But you are the one who has to know what these changes are, so you can continue to do the things you need to do to be independent."*

—Barbara Schrock, Ph.D.

Rationale for working hard in rehabilitation: plasticity

o *"Research tells us that chemistry in the brain changes with stimulation—so when we are doing rehab, we are not only compensating, but we are stimulating cells so they will sprout maximally."*

—Barbara Schrock, Ph.D.

Renegotiate your environment metaphor for compensatory strategies

o *"You're having some trouble with something we call executive function. This is how your brain makes plans, organizes time, prioritizes, pays attention, and solves complicated problems. What we need to do is help you renegotiate your environment, so you can work better. Right now we can't change your brain, but we can make changes to the environment so your brain can work better. Here's an example" (bring up things like block scheduling, etc.).*

—Susan McPherson, Ph.D.

o *"We need to set up the environment to be your frontal lobe, because the TBI has affected how well your frontal lobe is working. So, for example, we can color-code your calendar, and...."*

—Susan McPherson, Ph.D.

Creating realistic accommodations

Most people don't have enough power to change their work environment; their lives may not match your recommendations. Neuropsychologists need to go beyond recommending accommodations, and work collaboratively with patients to figure out how to create realistic work-arounds in their employment setting.

o *"If you are the boss, you can tell everyone not to interrupt you. Since you're not the boss, let's think about what you might be able to do instead."*

—*Karin McCoy, Ph.D.*

Joining with patients to facilitate use of compensatory strategies

Patients tend to hate "memory books" or notebooks; they feel like they are announcing to the world that there is something wrong with them. In contrast, people tend to love PDAs and smartphones. They key is to remind patients that everyone now uses these devices to help them be more organized and efficient.

o *"No one is going to know you have brain injury" (pull out own smartphone); "do you know how many times a day I pull this out?"*

—*Joseph H. Ricker, Ph.D.*

Opera metaphor for perspective on deficits

It's helpful to keep the feedback positive. As neuropsychologists, we can offer our perspective to help patients and families know that yes, they have a deficit, but it doesn't have to wreck their life.

o *"Look, you know you've got a memory problem. It's not going to get any worse. Your memory is not gone, it's just impaired. You need to compensate for it. You can appreciate the opera just the same as you've always done. You don't need new learning to enjoy your life."*

—*Christopher Randolph, Ph.D.*

EMOTIONAL ISSUES WITH ACQUIRED BRAIN INJURY RECOVERY

Following an acquired brain injury, many patients experience depression, heightened anxiety, poor social pragmatics, and interpersonal insensitivity. Catastrophic reactions can also occur in this context. Talking directly to the patient about these responses is not always as productive as working with family members or staff. It is particularly important to help the family to distinguish between depression and changes in cognitive or emotional systems that result in emotional flattening or irritability.

Post-TBI and -CVA depression can interfere with participation in rehabilitation activities, reintegration into the community, and family relationships. It is also miserable for patients. Explaining the possibility of developing depression may "inoculate" patients and their families, and can lead to more rapid treatment if the symptom emerges. Mild depression after TBI can also be reframed to patients and families as a good indicator of recovery. Emotional and social changes can also occur secondary to the brain injury itself (as opposed to emotional reaction to TBI or CVA). In these instances, it is very helpful to deal with patients' anxiety and guilt over their emotional changes, as many feel that their overblown reactions are their fault, or a sign of character weakness.

○ *For the general public in this post-Freudian era, whenever there are emotional changes, they will be attributed to psychological/behavioral issues. Therefore patients might say, "I don't know why I'm like this, I feel lousy."*

"The brain is the organ of thinking, and also feeling. You need to understand that brain injury can lead directly to emotional changes. Like depression, anxiety, impulsivity, or irritability. We might start to go off on our family members or friends. That also is a symptom of brain injury."

—*Tony Wong, Ph.D.*

Inoculating patients against depression

This approach is designed to "inoculate" patients against depressive feelings. Predicting some depression down the road can normalize the experience for patients and reduce associated guilt and feelings of isolation that often accompany depression. A point of caution is warranted, however, as an overly emphatic delivery could create a self-fulfilling prophecy.

○ *"I'm going to tell you—it's going to be rocky. You're going to continue to make progress, but it's going to be over a"* (gesture) *"looonger period of time. Over the next three months, you're going to notice that the honeymoon is over. You will find out who your friends really are. You will find some people who ask, 'Why aren't you just snapping out of it?' And there's a good chance you might get a little bummed out. I'm not trying to discourage you, but you've got to be prepared for the fact.*

You've made so much progress so far—your parents were told that 'your child might not survive'—so what do doctors know? So you have made—I've been doing this for 27 years—you've made very un-average progress. In fact, no offense, statistically speaking you should be dead. Now, I'm glad you're not! But all bets are off at this point. I can tell you that I've seen people like you who have done better than average and that it still wasn't a cakewalk. You will still have some problems down the road—and I just want to you to get that. Let's talk about how we are going to deal with that. Right now, your attitude is very good. You've got family support that is very good. It's a very good sign that you have that support. Right now, I don't think you need to see a counselor. But if that time comes, and I'm not saying for sure it will, but if that time comes, I want you to see someone."

—*Jacobus Donders, Ph.D.*

Explaining how antidepressants work

This is one way of explaining the use of therapy and medication together. It's not an "either or."

○ *"You're going to have some changes in your mood. Instead of the changes being this big"* (wide hand gesture), *"medication kind of boxes it in so it doesn't get out of control" (narrower hand gesture). "It's still not a happy pill. You're still going to have to deal with the stress. That's what therapy is for."*

—Jacobus Donders, Ph.D.

Connection between improving awareness and depression

o *"We just did retesting. You know a lot of your test scores are improving. Memory has gotten better, and attention has gotten better. And processing is better. But you're looking more depressed, or more anxious since the last time we tested. We do see this a lot—sometimes people get depressed as they are recovering and become more aware of the problems they are having. As you become more aware, this mild depression might actually be a sign of recovery. What do you think of that?"*

—Joseph H. Ricker, Ph.D.

Explaining apathy

Apathy is an underappreciated aspect of brain injury and neurological disease; it's often not understood or discussed enough. Even though the two major dimensions underlying personality change after a TBI are apathy and disinhibition, disinhibition gets more attention for obvious reasons. But apathy can be very difficult for families as well.

o *"This is a neurological syndrome. This is not like normal sadness, or the 'I don't care,' that you or I would experience. It looks like depression, but the difference is that when people are depressed, they are hurting, and they are sad, and they are feeling their emotions in a negative and painful way. The problem with apathy is not that you experience negative emotions—it's that you don't feel any emotions in the same way. You don't feel the highs—or the lows. Nothing bothers these patients much. They don't get touched or moved. When they hear someone is dying or sick, it's not that they don't care, it's that they can't care. They can't get to their feelings. Usually it's a truncation of emotions. The negatives don't bother them as much, but they don't feel the positives as much either. They don't feel joy; not to that intensity. It can be severe, where people don't feel anything—or just mild. When it's more severe, they are not feeling their emotions. Everyone may think they are depressed. But they're not.*

"Besides emotions, apathy also effects thinking and actions. In severe cases, there's no initiation at all. People will just sit there and won't get up and get going. Most importantly, they don't even have goal-directed thought. When you ask them what they are thinking about, and they say, 'Nothing,' that's true! Their minds are literally just blank."

—Jim Irby, Ph.D.

Spiritual reflection to improve mood

A helpful focus during feedback session for patients who have survived a severe TBI or stroke is how blessed they are to be alive. People tend to appreciate it. They have all kinds of other pulmonary problems, spinal, cardiac dissections, orthopedic. They are still a mess. They know it. They are overcoming huge obstacles—it's no secret. Focusing on the spiritual aspect of their survival can be a positive motivating component. The biggest challenge we face is the despair, hopelessness, and depression that may ensue for people who suffer this horrible trauma. Saying I'm not the most religious person is an understatement. I come from a long line of atheists and agnostics. It's not easy for me to resonate with many people's religious leanings. I try to focus on the blessed nature of their being a living person—this seems helpful. When given an opening, many will naturally start to describe their religious leanings.

   o *"Gee, as we all know, it's really lucky you are still alive."*
                                                            —*Robert M. Bilder, Ph.D.*

Explaining catastrophic reactions

   o *"What your father is experiencing, pretty regularly, is what we call a 'catastrophic reaction.' This is common after stroke, and should improve over time. Before the stroke, he did well under busy or mildly stressful conditions. But now he is likely to get overwhelmed. While he is recovering, he is not going to have a lot of insight into this. So really, we can think about the conditions around him as creating the problem. Keep the situation around your father less stimulating, less overwhelming. Don't take him to the mall or shopping center for the time being."*
                                                            —*David E. Tupper, Ph.D.*

Differentiating pseudobulbar affect and depression

   o *"The right side of the brain seems to be more dominant in terms of emotional regulation. I want to reassure you that you are not a basket case. This is part of the stroke. All those pathways that were affected by your stroke run right through the emotional systems. You can have a hair trigger on tears. Little things just bring those tears up—and that's not how you were before the stroke. The way you know it's lability and not depression, is because if you change the subject, the tears dry up immediately. You know it's a threshold issue. It's not that you are deeply sad. It's that any topic that has any connection to your heartstrings makes you tear up. You can say 'family' and people will tear up. It doesn't mean you are sad, or depressed."*
                                                            —*Barbara Schrock, Ph.D.*

Light switch metaphor for post-stroke emotional changes

   o *"Sometimes, after these types of strokes, a person may laugh or cry out of nowhere. And you ask them, 'Is there anything upsetting you or is this coming out of nowhere?' Because sometimes with CVA, especially right middle cerebral artery CVA, it's like a switch, where anything that has an emotional content switches things to laughing or crying without necessarily being linearly related to the degree of emotional experience a person is having." (Turning to the patient's family,) "I just asked your father, 'Have you seen your grandson yet?' This doesn't have to be a particularly emotional question, but it just flipped that switch to tears."*

—Joel Rosenbaum, Ph.D.

o   *It's important to realize that when people have these strokes they tend to talk more slowly and cry more often. They tend to have a flattening of affect that is directly related to their stroke. It looks like depression, but may not be depression. It is important to ask them if they feel depressed. Or if they get tearful, ask them, "Is there something you are thinking that is making you feel tearful?" This gives you a better sense of whether they are sad.*

—Joel Rosenbaum, Ph.D.

Explaining shallow irritability

o   *"Some little thing that wouldn't have bothered you before—suddenly sets you off, 'Kapow!' Zero to 60. You lose your temper! A few minutes later, it's over for you— but everyone else is shell-shocked." (Patient and family members are nodding.) "That's different from depression. It's a little impulse-control issue. It happens to many people in the beginning after a stroke. This is very common. It's not depression. It's likely to happen more often if you are tired; it's the same thing we all experience once in a while. It's a threshold issue though, and it takes almost nothing to trigger it now."*

—Barbara Schrock, Ph.D.

Anger management following CVA

o   *"After a stroke, it can be much harder to control anger. The anger can just get out of control. As soon as you notice that you are getting angry, I'm going to tell you something you can do to reduce that anger and get back in control. But in case you don't notice, someone else might, and they can help you with this.*

"If someone starts to lose control, anyone can say, 'Time out!' The goal at that moment in time is not to resolve the issue. Rather it is to get under control. Without the influence of the frontal lobes, your behavior is controlled by the impulse or stimuli in front of your face. If the impulse is anger, the stimulus might be your wife. So the goal is to get away from the stimulus. Come back and discuss it later. The earlier you notice your temper getting out of control, the greater chance you have of controlling it. It gets better with time, and if it doesn't, then there are some medications that can help."

—Barbara Schrock, Ph.D.

Explaining mirroring of emotions

o *"Sometimes with frontal or right Middle Cerebral Artery (MCA) syndrome, patients can get stuck mirroring; they mirror your emotions. They may be 'stimulus bound.' If you come in and approach them in a very concerned way, they will reflect that emotion. You may unwittingly hold them in that emotional state, limiting their abilities to participate in a different way. You need to be able to switch emotional tones; you may need to be more upbeat. You may need to be able to switch topics to one less emotionally laden so that the individual figuratively and physically can breathe and not be so bogged down with emotion."*

—*Joel Rosenbaum, Ph.D.*

Emotional Flattening

o *Oftentimes, a lot of people tell me that what they experience is a sense of emotional distancing—almost apathy. "I wish I cared but I don't." It's not a psychiatric issue; it's a part of the stroke.*

—*Barbara Schrock, Ph.D.*

Discussing the emotional impact of ABI on the spouse and family

During feedback, it is helpful to foreshadow post-stroke depression while discussing issues of recovery. It is also very helpful, with the permission of the patient, to discuss potential depression with his or her spouse—and to find out what their own concerns are. Does the patient's spouse feel they are handling the increased burden well? Are *they* feeling depressed or overwhelmed? This conversation can lead the neuropsychologist to recommend community or family resources. A lot of this has historically been the purview of social work. It would be easy to push things off on the social workers or physicians. But with the type of information we know about the CVA's effect on day-to-day functioning on the whole family, it takes a lot of steps out of the equations; we know how the patient will cognitively interact with the services. In this context, many neuropsychologists will invite their patients to call when problems arise, taking on a case-management role, with their unique neuropsychological perspective. This can preclude the development of other issues.

o *"I want to take some time to talk about how you are both experiencing all of these changes from an emotional perspective...."*

—*Joseph H. Ricker, Ph.D.*

Talking with spouses about separating from patients with emotional dyscontrol

Following severe TBI, a patient's personality changes might create more significant, even terrible change in their family's life. Anger issues, unawareness of deficits, and disinhibition can create an abusive context for the spouse and children. This is meant to be directed to a spouse who expresses the need to leave the patient, in a separate feedback session:

> o *"I have known wives who have spent years hanging in there with this unpleasantly difficult situation. They have been scared to death about what the family would say if they left. Once they made the break, a sister-in-law or mother-in-law would say, 'I don't know why you stayed so long.' I also add, and may repeat several times over, that separation does not mean abandonment; and should the spouse seem ready to make a move, I recommend that they find an appropriate living situation for the patient, and keep a close and continuing contact with the patient and whoever is giving the patient care. I also remind them that, should they make the change, patients can be reassured of spending holidays and other times with the family—they are not cut off and not abandoned."*
> —Muriel D. Lezak, Ph.D.

EXPLAINING SPECIFIC NEUROLOGICAL, COGNITIVE, AND BEHAVIORAL SEQUELAE OF CVA

Feedback in stroke populations must be pitched to the patient's age and lifespan stage. For example, with young adults, returning to work and parenting issues are often prominent concerns. The cause of the CVA is often a vasospasm or a burst aneurysm, as opposed to the typical stroke that comes later in life with plenty of warning (e.g., after a 30-year history of hypertension or diabetes). This means the stroke literally hits young adults out of the blue. On the other hand, when stroke affects older patients, caregiving issues can be particularly problematic, especially when spouses have their own physical or cognitive difficulties. Childhood stroke brings its own host of difficulties, although most of the discussion points are similar to those for other acquired brain injuries (consequently, readers are referred to Chapter 13, "Neurological Disorders," for pearls relating to pediatric CVA).

Focal symptoms are generally easier to explain to patients and families, particularly with the help of brain models as props; patients and family members tend to "get" an aphasia, visual neglect, or hemiparesis. It can be more challenging to help patients understand the source and consequences of general slowing and executive dysfunction (see also Chapter 7, "Attention Deficit Hyperactivity Disorder," which provides a number of applicable executive-function and slowed-processing pearls). Finally, many CVA patients also have difficulty appreciating the bigger picture of how their deficits will affect their daily life, even if they do not have a classic anosognosia. Knowing how to explain a patient's deficits in applied terms can often make it real enough for them to both accept and work around their problems.

Ten men carrying a log metaphor for stroke

> o *"You have 10 men carrying a heavy log. A couple of them get injured and leave. Then you have eight men left carrying the log. At first it's hard, but eventually they get stronger and stronger, and then they can carry the log again. But sometimes,*

you get a situation in which eight of the ten men get injured and leave. Then you only have two men carrying the log. If that happens, the remaining men have to get a lot stronger before they can carry the log again, and so it can take a long time to get to that point. But, even when the men get as strong as they can, the log may still need to be carried more slowly, and by the end of the day the men may get very tired. And of course, in the situation in which all the men get injured— there are no men left to carry the log. In those situations, function is not going to return."

—*Yana Suchy, Ph.D.*

Memory board metaphor for thalamic stroke

With a thalamic stroke, there tends to be a dense learning deficit, but everything else may look pretty good.

o *"Your MRI scan shows that this is a thalamic stroke. It's like having a bad sector on your computer's memory board. Unlike a computer, we can't go in and replace the memory board, but we can use a patch. For example, using this smartphone can help."*

—*Susan McPherson Ph.D.*

Explaining aperceptive agnosias

o *"He has something we call 'aperceptive agnosia.' It's not that he is blind, it's just that he can't make sense of what he sees. It's a little bit like trying to watch HBO without having subscribed to it. The image is there, but it's scrambled. You kind of see it- but it's hard to understand what you are looking at when it's not very clear."*

—*Yana Suchy, Ph.D.*

APHASIAS

It always helps to normalize the patient's symptoms: "This is not just your weakness; this symptom makes complete sense given the location of the stroke."

o *"Of course your language is not so good—even if I hadn't tested you, given the location of the stroke, we could have predicted that these would have been the areas of difficulty.…"*

—*Barbara Schrock, Ph.D.*

I never see an aphasic patient alone for feedback; I always bring in the family. Very often you have people that can fool family members or staff into believing they comprehend more than they do.

o *"A lot of this may go over your head because of comprehension problems. But I will give a big overview of this picture. You fool people! You are good at it. But it's really important that you and your family know that you are not getting all the information. Here is one way you can check it out." (Turn to spouse,) "You can say, 'Tell me in your own words what I just said.' It's also important, when going to doctor appointments or whatever, that you bring someone along so you get all the important information."*

—Barbara Schrock, Ph.D.

Assessing comprehension of feedback with expressive aphasics

When patients have aphasia, feedback can be particularly challenging, especially if you want to validate their understanding of what you are sharing. If the patient has good receptive language, but has difficulty with expressive language, you should avoid open-ended questions when assessing their comprehension. Instead, use yes and no questions. When possible, start with the most general aspect of the question and work toward the more specific aspects, not vice-versa.

o *"Mr. Smith, do you understand what I just said?" (Not, "What is your understanding of what I just said?" Or, "Can you let me know what you think about this?")*

—Joel Rosenbaum, Ph.D.

EXPLAINING SPECIFIC NEUROLOGICAL, COGNITIVE, AND BEHAVIORAL SEQUELAE OF MODERATE AND SEVERE TBI

Often, following a TBI, family members have a tough time coping with the patient's increased impulsivity and lack of judgment, particularly because the patient *looks* just the same as they always have on the outside. Furthermore, due to the acquired executive dysfunction, patients may be so variable with their capacities that there is general confusion about what they can and cannot accomplish. Sharing neuropsychological data can be an effective way to connect the dots for families between changes in behavior and personality, and changes to the brain from the TBI.

Helping patients understand their cognitive and behavioral changes is also important, and often done best with props. Many clinicians will use a traditional desktop 3D model. Neuropsychologists are also beginning to use iPads or other tablets for patient education (the iPad has several free applications available with fully interactive brain models). For the younger set—seeing the neuropsychologist's explanation accompanied with a model on a tablet, has more cachet; it is cooler than a plastic model, and like anything with a screen, might hold their attention longer. Of course, neuropsychologists also have a host of metaphors that further demonstrate their points.

Tipped bookshelf metaphor for post-TBI brain changes

It helps to have asked about patients' premorbid hobbies and activities in the initial clinical interview so this pearl can be tailored to the patients' specific interests.

o *"Before you had this TBI you were who you were. You were into hockey. Everything you know about hockey is on the top shelf. Your brain is like this really, really,*

really tall bookshelf, with hundreds of thousands of books. On the next shelf are books about girls and dating, then basketball, then math.

"What happens with a TBI is your bookshelf gets tipped over. And the books get scattered. Depending on the severity, the books might get really scattered. As part of rehab, your bookshelf gets straightened up. Most of the books get put back on the right shelf. And your intelligence hasn't been affected. But some of your books are upside down and sideways, or on the wrong shelf. That's why when you go to say your sister's name, you can't find it. It's on a different shelf. Or when you want a math fact, you have to really think. And it's either going to go back all on its own, or you will have to relearn some things. The content is still there. But it's an access problem."

—*Michael Joschko, Ph.D.*

Using imaging results in feedback sessions

Sometimes, neuropsychologists are the first ones to explain what happened to the patient from the brain injury. In many rehabilitation hospitals, each patient room, as well as clinician offices, have a dedicated monitor to show people their scans. If appropriate, and cleared with the attending to make sure one is not stepping on toes (and they are generally more than happy to have the neuropsychologist spend an hour talking to the patient), the injury characteristics can be explained.

People are fascinated to see their own brains. And family members tend to like it. I have a few rules of thumb when considering reviewing scans with patients: Never review a scan cold with a patient; always go through the scan first with the radiology report at your elbow. You need to understand the scan prior to talking about it. If there is something really goofy, or if something is evident that is not in the report ("July phenomena"—first-year radiology residents), any conflicts should be cleared up behind the scenes. This maintains the patient's trust that everyone is on the same page.

It is often helpful to bring imaging in when the person doesn't seem to accept they had an injury to the brain. Parents of college students who are not getting it that their child had a significant brain injury particularly benefit from seeing the imaging. Some break down crying when the reality hits that they really did have a significant injury.

o *"This is what happened to you. This area here is called a subarachnoid hemorrhage. Your brain bled. See, this is what happened in your brain."*

—*Joseph H. Ricker, Ph.D.*

o *"These regions of the brain are very involved in being able to control emotions. They also work in planning, judgment, picking up on social cues, and monitoring internal emotional states. When there is damage to those areas, these things become dysregulated." (If there is a scan finding, at that point, go back to the imaging): "See that frontal contusion?"*

—*Erin D. Bigler, Ph.D.*

Organ of thinking metaphor for explaining TBI

o *"Just like the liver is the organ of metabolism, and the stomach is the organ of digestion, your brain is your organ of thinking. Different parts of the brain do different things as far as thinking, and for schoolwork and work endeavors."* (Make it very matter of fact.) *"This is what happened in the brain to you."*

—Joseph H. Ricker, Ph.D.

Explaining axonal damage

o *"There are these special fibers in the brain that carry messages over relatively long distances. They are covered by these special insulating sheaths that allow the messages to be carried even faster, and enable the communication at high speed across the brain. And sometimes those fibers can be damaged."*

—Robert M. Bilder, Ph.D.

Acknowledging obvious deficits

o *In the beginning, with TBI patients, I hardly say anything more than:* "Well, your memory is not so hot, but you already knew that."

—Barbara Schrock, Ph.D.

The Christmas time in the mall effect metaphor for tbi

In inpatient rehabilitation settings, an important aspect of feedback is educating the family about the disorganizing effects of overstimulation on the patient's behavior.

o *"One of things that can overload an injured brain is too much going on around them for too long. I call this the 'Christmastime in the mall effect.' You know how you go shopping in the mall at Christmastime and you're really exhausted and cranky after a couple of hours even though all you've been doing is walking around? It's because they have the tall ceilings and open floor plans, noise is bouncing around, it's bright and people are all doing their own thing. It's chaos. After a while, you're tired of it, and you just kind of want it all to go away, right?*

"Having a brain injury means that your family member is not going to be in control over his/her attention. You and I can narrow our attention and pull it into a tight beam, putting it where we want it, but if I stop talking, you can also broaden it out and hear the noises outside this office, the air, and feel that tag tickling at the back of your neck. Because someone with a brain injury isn't in control over their attention, they are either going to be sucked into something, like the TV, or going to be wide open and taking everything in all at once. They're feeling everything, tasting everything, smelling everything, seeing everything, and hearing everything

all at once. They can't screen anything out, so it's like they're living in the mall at Christmastime 24–7, and they can't leave. You can imagine how that feels. You'd be cranky, too.

"Those things that you've been seeing, the restlessness, the irritability, impulsivity, withdrawal, and zoning out, are all signs of overstimulation, that there's been too much going on for too long. So, we're going to need to be very careful about how much is going on around your family member. Until your family member is more in control of their own brains, we're going to need to keep everything around them very low-key, calm, slow, and quiet, with nice long rest breaks in between."

—*Anne Bradley, Ph.D.*

MILD TRAUMATIC BRAIN INJURY

Because the prognosis for recovery from mild traumatic brain injury (mTBI) is very good, it is important to reassure patients. When patients are seen shortly after a mild traumatic brain injury, expectations for a complete recovery should be set as early as possible. This can also be said during the initial consultation, as a way of foreshadowing the feedback session. Some patients have been given incorrect information from other medical professionals, which reflect outdated research and clinical lore about an expected poor prognosis. For example, patients may have been encouraged to seek disability from work, or psychotherapy with the goal of "mourning their loss" of cognitive function, following a concussion. They may therefore be initially skeptical about hearing about their lack of permanent damage. At times the feedback sessions may resemble those of somatoform patients where a tug of war needs to be avoided between perspectives of health and illness. (Refer to the "Somatoform" chapter for strategies to acknowledge the presence of real difficulties with daily cognitive function caused by factors other than brain damage).

Explaining mTBI physiology

Patients commonly ask, "Where in the brain is the concussion?"

o *"Concussion, or this form of mild brain injury, is really a diffuse injury at a cellular level. It's not like I can say, 'Because you had a blow to the front of your head, that's where the concussion is.' It's really at a cellular level. In your case it's likely that those cells were stretched and didn't function normally for a time, but those cells weren't killed. They aren't dead."*

—*Michael McCrea, Ph.D.*

o *(While showing a picture of the brain,) "These fibers can be stretched, bruised, sloshed around, and this is where the initial symptoms come from. You may experience a variety of symptoms in the recovery stage that may seem odd to you. You might experience a variety of thinking and other problems" (try to normalize it).*

—*Munro Cullum Ph.D.*

SETTING THE EXPECTATION FOR RECOVERY WITH MTBI

> o *"We really don't expect to see much. We're just doing this testing to make sure."*
> *(Then at feedback,) "People after this type of injury recover completely. In a few*
> *weeks, you will be back to 100 percent."*
> —Bill Barr, Ph.D.

> o *"Good news—I know you had this traumatic experience—you were shook up for a*
> *while and had these scary symptoms. Everything we have seen indicates you are on*
> *a typical recovery path and you should be back to your old self."*
> —Robert M. Bilder, Ph.D.

Counseling mTBI patients who have been given misinformation by other professionals

Other specialties, (e.g., occupational therapy, physical therapy, medicine), are often giving information that is directly opposite to what we know—like referring to brain injury as a unitary concept; mTBI is really a separate issue. Patients hear advice to "Stay cocooned"; they might hear that they face a long, unpredictable recovery; and they are often given the concept of "mourning your loss." A neuropsychologist's role has to include patient education. Including scientific evidence as part of this is powerful.

> o *"Listen, I don't expect you to buy into this 100 percent. If I were you, I might not*
> *either. Let's look at what's going on here. You've been followed for two years. I've*
> *seen the records. Every professional has told you for two years that you have diffuse*
> *brain injury. You can't work. I am going to tell you something different than what*
> *you've heard. I'm going to show you the evidence base." (I have a computer in the*
> *room where feedback is given and show PowerPoint slides including data from the*
> *NCAA study.) "Have any of the doctors that have treated you talked to you about*
> *the evidence base?" ("No.") "You are going to have to decide. Look at your test*
> *data. This is evidence too." (I usually give test data first, then the slide show). "If*
> *you can at least just open the door in your head, that there may be something here*
> *you can control. Why don't you just give this a try? Give it a shot."*
> —Dominic Carone Ph.D.

After hearing compelling data that they are in fact completely recovered from their mild traumatic brain injury, patients can feel angry: "All these people have told me it's brain damage all these years!"

> o *"Even doctors have misconceptions with this. But if you look at the research studies,*
> *it is clear that a concussion does not have lasting effects."*
> —Bill Barr, Ph.D.

Vicious cycle metaphor for mtbi recovery

I have an 8 x 11 blowup of Michael McCrea's JAMA article "Recovery Curves of Athletes" that I show patients before I say this.

o *"This is the typical recovery course for a mild traumatic brain injury. Almost all of the physiological stuff is over in the first week. And by the end of the first month, it's definitely over. People recover entirely by this point here. So, three months down the road from the injury, the physiological changes in the brain are done, and what we are left with, when symptoms continue, are stressors that have taken over. Let me explain how it works with an example:*

"Everyone has headaches. When you get a headache, you say, 'Okay, I've got a headache, am I stressed?' But if you've had a mild brain injury, it's easy to freak out, thinking, 'Oh no! The TBI is back!' And that causes increased stress, tense muscles, and the headache worsens. When you've got a really bad headache, and your stress at the thought of being brain-damaged goes way up again, it becomes a vicious cycle."

—Bill Barr, Ph.D.

ATHLETES AND mTBI

The way athletes, coaches, parents, professional sports franchises, and medical professionals think about concussions has changed continuously in the past few decades. Years ago, the consensus was that concussions were just "dings." And athletes were given implicit or explicit instructions to "get up and shake it off." With increasing recognition of the potential long-term effects of multiple concussions, many more athletes are referred for neuropsychological assessment following concussion. That said, biases to return to play as soon as possible continue to be held by players, coaches, and parents, and can make discussions in feedback difficult. A teenagers' general feeling of invincibility, of course, does not help.

Gas tank metaphor for mTBI recovery in athletes

o *"This is what I'm going to tell your parents. You just had a concussion. Now if you had just had a single concussion, we probably wouldn't be having this conversation. You've had several in a row, and you didn't have complete recovery in between. That's why you have begun to have headaches at school. I know how important football is to you. I don't pretend to know what it feels like—because I don't. But I also know you want to go to college and become a doctor"* (or whatever.) *"You not only need to use those great hands of yours"* (wide receiver), *"you also need your brain. With every concussion you kill off a few brain cells, and we can all do that because we are all born with a few extra brain cells. We've got a reserve in the tank. But your tank is either empty—or you've dipped too far into your tank. My concern is that if you get another concussion like this it will set you back even further. Now we aren't talking just about you not playing football. We are talking about not being able to go to college anymore."* (To parents): *"If it were my kid I would be very nervous about him going back. You can probably get someone to say it's okay. But if it were my kid I would say, 'Enough!' You've only got one brain. But think about it—how many people play in the NFL? You will need your brain for the rest of your life."*

—Jacobus Donders, Ph.D.

Cautioning against further concussions

o *"What you're experiencing now is normal. It's normal to be a little bit irritable. Normal to have a headache. The typical recovery time is short—a few weeks. You were in good shape before; you're going to be fine. In the meantime though, you don't want to do anything stupid. And what is stupid? Getting another concussion. Now, you are wrestling, let's talk about it.... This is not the time to be bungee jumping. That doesn't mean you have to be a hermit. You can go out with your friends...."*
—*Jacobus Donders, Ph.D.*

o *"He's got seven concussions. In my experience, after seven, number eight comes easily. You should think about that."*
—*Bill Barr, Ph.D.*

Feedback with professional athletes

The issue of sports-related concussions has received a lot more attention, and has intensified recently. You have high-profile football players with a history of concussions who are reportedly developing syndromes akin to amoytrophic lateral sclerosis (ALS) or Alzheimer disease. Now it's gotten into many athletes' knowledge base that it's possible that "if I let myself in for enough of these injuries it could have a nightmarish outcome down the road." Neuropsychologists are one part of the post-concussion and return-to-play process. One goal of feedback is to try to educate and empower the player, because the pressure is coming from the team—and from their DNA to get back to competition and contact.

o *"I don't need to see you again. From a neuropsychological perspective, your performance on my cognitive tests indicates that you are good to go. However, you are describing persisting problems with insomnia, dizziness, and light sensitivity. So, ultimately return to play should not happen until those symptoms have resolved completely. You are fine to return from a cognitive perspective. But here's the deal. Until these other symptoms are resolved, you should not be putting yourself in a position to absorb further contact. It's really your call."*
—*Aaron Nelson, Ph.D.*

REFERENCE

Grace J, Malloy PF. *Frontal Systems Behavior Scale Professional Manual.* Lutz, FL: Psychological Assessment Resources; 2001.

13 Neurological Disorders

(Countinued)

CANCER, MULTIPLE SCLEROSIS, genetic disorders, seizures, and other disorders affecting cognition are included in this chapter. Many of the feedback techniques are disease-specific. Others can be used more broadly.

CANCER

In the distress of an initial cancer diagnosis and treatment, family members and patients may have been told, but not fully processed, key information. In the context of a neuro-oncology service, neuropsychologists are often the clinicians who see the patient for the longest span of time. Neuropsychologists have the time therefore, to explain the impact of the illness in understandable terms. Neuropsychological feedback sessions become an opportunity to ask what the radiation oncology team has told families, and then to provide and discuss information again in a collaborative manner.

The goals of feedback are dependent on the stage of treatment and the nature of the cancer. Early in treatment, the neuropsychologist may primarily engage in developing a relationship with the family; introducing their role in the long-term care of the patient. Subsequent feedback sessions tend to focus on the effects of lesions and secondary effects of treatment on cognition. The "psychologist" in neuropsychologist is particularly relevant in these cases, as clinicians must be mindful of the extraordinary stressors patients and their family systems are experiencing. The relief of having their loved one alive may lead to a lack of focus on residual cognitive changes and upcoming hurdles for returning to work or school.

The neuropsychologist's role on the neuro-oncology team

During feedback sessions, it is important to reintroduce who you are and what your role is, particularly as in hospital-based work, new players often show up in feedback sessions. Families may be so overwhelmed that the first time you spoke with them, they didn't process this information.

o *"I'm Dr. Janzen. I'm the neuropsychologist with the neuro-oncology team (Drs. X, Y, and Z that you've met). My role is to help you understand the impact the brain tumor and treatment has on your child's learning and thinking abilities. How she makes sense of what she sees and what she hears, her attention and memory. And how all of those things affect how she learns at school: reading, and math and writing. We're here to get a sense of your child's strengths and weaknesses in those areas and to give you some information about what we might expect in the future."*

—Laura Janzen, Ph.D.

o *"I know right now this doesn't seem like an important thing in your life, because your child is here. It's so early, and you all are so scared. Over time my role will become more important and we will work more closely together. A year from now I will probably be someone you are thinking of—after all this part is done and you're back to a normal life again with your child in school and you're working with them on homework. If you're noticing some of the things we've talked about, that's when you want to be in touch."*

—Laura Janzen, Ph.D.

o *"My job is to be the 'worst-case scenario girl.' To pick up on every single possible thing that could go wrong or that your child is at risk for. And to come up with intervention plans to avoid the risk as much as possible, or to bolster skills so there is not a major skill deficit. So I found these five things: let's go through what these things are, and then prioritize what to work on first."*

—Jennifer Turek Queally, Ph.D.

Cancer treatments' effects on cognition

Clinicians might launch into accurate technical explanations, but these often don't stick. Families or patients might come out of a conversation with a pediatric neurosurgeon and say to the neuropsychologist, "What is it they are planning to do?" It is helpful to supplement those technical conversations with an explanation that is simple and includes an analogy.

o *"All cancers are fast-growing cells. Radiation therapy works by disrupting or destroying the DNA. That's the instructional set for how a cell replicates itself. Then, when the tumor cells try to replicate they can't because the radiation has gotten rid of their instruction set. The problem is that the radiation doesn't know the difference between a good cell and a cancer cell. So developmentally, when good cells start to replicate, children can have deficits that they didn't have initially, because the radiation has also gotten rid of the instructions for the good cells."*

—Jim Scott, Ph.D.

In the acute moment of the horror of the diagnosis and treatment, the only focus is preserving life. Sometimes there are decisions to be made about such things as different levels of radiation or chemotherapy. The parents' ability to comprehensively evaluate information and make a decision in the moment can be superficial. Many parents walk out thinking—"I chose not to have radiation; my kid will be fine."

We can't get around the fact that treatments for brain tumors kill off developing cells—that's the whole point of receiving chemotherapy and radiation. In the middle of child development, we have a lot of rapidly developing cells. We have to treat the brain, and we know that this changes how the cells are developing. Some kids are more at risk for learning issues. Kids who are treated under age three are at higher risk. Girls often have more long-lasting, late effects.

o *"Your nine-year-old girl, who was diagnosed at age two, had to have a lot of treatment. She overcame tremendous odds by beating cancer at the age of two. That also means that there will be late effects. Just like you look out for and monitor cardiac effects, there are certain things we will monitor for, like cognitive and learning issues. And there are some things that you are seeing—that's why you are here."*

—*Jennifer Turek Queally, Ph.D.*

Introducing the long-term effects of radiation is a challenge. People might not be ready to face the news early on. Many have a vague sense that something bad might happen, but tend to fall back on, "We don't care, we're happy our kid's alive, and what we see now will get better, right?"

This is a hard conversation to have, and it will probably need to occur over and over. This is the first introduction. Families hear this initially but it often doesn't sink in, not until the effects start to emerge. Not until kids have returned to school, sometimes a year after the initial diagnosis—that's when it becomes evident. The key thing is to develop a relationship so the parents know that the neuropsychologist is the go-to person for these things.

> o *"Radiation specifically damages the white matter of the brain. White matter is the fatty coating or sheath that goes around the nerve cells and helps areas of the brain communicate with one another. The main thing we see is that transmission of information becomes slower. There can be problems with attention, and overall a slower rate of learning. We won't see those effects for maybe a year or even more. And it varies from one child to another. Children tend to be more at risk because those parts of the brain aren't fully developed at the time of the treatment. It's hard to predict the effect for any one child, and that's why we are going to do some testing now to see where your child is at. Over time we will be redoing this to see what changes have occurred and try to support you in dealing with any difficulties."*
>
> —*Laura Janzen, Ph.D.*

Discussing the effects of neurosurgery

Sometimes it's clear that the neurosurgical intervention has affected cognition. The neurosurgeon might have to cut through normal tissue to insert multiple shunts. Sometimes you think, "Well, what we are seeing is partly neurosurgical." But we have an obligation to be careful about not conveying to patients, "I think this damage is due to the neurosurgery," because the only reason that neurosurgery happened was because of the tumor. It's important not to inadvertently "blame" the surgeon, because the surgery was necessary. They did what they had to do to get rid of the tumor. I try to be thoughtful about how to present the effects as an entire package coming from the tumor and the surgery.

> o *"Because of the tumor, your child needed neurosurgery—it was essential, right?"* (*They nod.*) *"Because of what's happened, now we are seeing these cognitive effects. These areas of the brain, their functions have been affected. And this is what we are seeing."*
>
> —*Laura Janzen, Ph.D.*

Explaining the range of possible outcomes following pediatric cancer—"we don't have all the answers"

By the time families meet with neuropsychologists, they have heard survival numbers from the neuroradiologists. "Your child has XY chance of surviving five years." Sometimes families ask similar questions about other aspects of their child's outcome. "What's the likelihood, in numbers, that my child will go to college?" Or, "What is the percentage chance that my child will have cognitive decline?"

> o *"We know from years of research now that children who are treated earlier, before the age of three, and before school age, are at increased risk of having cognitive decline related to treatment. Girls appear to have more difficulty than boys over the long term. It has to do with the types of treatment required, like the dose, and the areas of the brain treated, but a lot of it we don't know. Some depends on how the tumor behaves. Recurrence requires more treatment and that makes the likelihood of cognitive problems higher. I can't give you numbers the way the other doctors have given you numbers because it is so individual. But also because there are opportunities at many points to intervene and provide supports and services. We don't know the ultimate outcome, but we will do everything we can to improve the outcome."*
> —*Laura Janzen, Ph.D.*

Under-attribution vs. over-attribution regarding a child's illness

As soon as their child is diagnosed, parents can become over-protective. They don't want their child to experience any failure. They coddle him and don't let him stretch his wings. Or, they might do the opposite. They are intent on letting their child have a totally normal experience: soccer, everything. But this might inadvertently expose their child to failure after failure.

> o *"It's important to let the child experience success and failure. A lot of times parents feel that every time their child has a temper tantrum, it must be the chemotherapy. And really, we might not know. It doesn't matter because you have to do the same things to fix it. Whether it's just a temper tantrum or the chemo. That might be behavior modification or other methods that we can talk about."*
> —*Jim Scott, Ph.D.*

Planning a return to school after long-term cancer treatment

This conversation helps them see that, "yes, we are in this terrible situation now, but there is a future. Life will return to normal. You will return to a job. Your child will return to school. And there will need to be lead-time."

> o *"Right now you are in the midst of intense treatment. But let's start thinking of when your child will return to school. Once they finish the bone marrow transplant, then we add three months where they will need homeschooling because of immunosupression. Then given everything we know about the course of treatment, your*

child would return the following September. The school will need some time to plan, so, let's think about a reasonable time to reassess, to prepare for a school meeting."
—Laura Janzen, Ph.D.

Focusing on the child's strengths in the context of acquired cognitive deficits

A child who had made it through a life-threatening illness became a seminal moment in my career. Year after year, some families come back for cognitive assessments, hearing "bad news" about their child's residual deficits, and they forget what they actually have, because that's not what we focus on. "This is low, that is impaired" … and they end up being really discouraged. But everyone wants their kid to be happy, and that is nearly always possible. In this one instance, I engaged the family in a little higher-level abstraction about their situation.

> o *"You don't like being here. I know: It's always the same bad news. Well, let's think about what you want. Look, he's saved. He's been saved. And he's been harmed by the disease, but you have your son, and you're going to have him. So what do you want for him?" (Parents reply, "We want him to graduate from high school, we want him to be happy.") "Well, you have that. You've got that."*

They said what they wanted for him. And I said, "He's got that." That ended up being the moment where the problem that had consumed all of their foreground attention for years finally began shifting to the background.
—Steve Hughes, Ph.D.

Mood Issues with Pediatric Neuro-Oncology

> o *"Based on everything you told me in the interview, and based on the information we got from the teacher and other professionals, it seems that there are some mood issues for your child. He seems unhappy" (describe symptoms): "these are things that wouldn't be unusual in a child who is coping with all he has had to. The good news is that there are treatments that can help your child feel better. Let's talk about a referral to a psychologist. We need to think about seeking that at our hospital versus in your community. Many treatments for mood issues require intensive work—biweekly. Is it possible for you to come here? We have psychologists who specialize in children's cancer and really understand those issues. But it may not be feasible for you all to come multiple times a week."*
> *—Laura Janzen, Ph.D.*

Sprint vs. Marathon Metaphor for Parents during their Child's Treatment for Cancer

> o *"You're going to be entering a marathon. You've been in this sprint section because you are dealing with a new diagnosis and it's overwhelming. You're working very*

hard just to cope and manage. But this is a long-term process. It's going to be a marathon for you. Here are the supports—this is what's available. Part of it is thinking ahead to save your energy for down the road. This is a long-term challenge."

—*Laura Janzen, Ph.D.*

When the cancer is terminal

When an adult patient's prognosis is terminal, a discussion of deficits becomes less important than a discussion of what the patient is still able to do.

o *"The neuropsychological tests showed some problems that you already knew about. Definitely, the problems are there. But your cognitive skills are still good. It's important to do all of your activities around the house. Go to your kid's gymnastic and tennis meets. Stay active, keep exercising your mental abilities. That helps things."*

—*Erin D. Bigler, Ph.D.*

GENETIC DISORDERS

Disclosing XY variants to schools

Many parents are hesitant to tell schools when their child has an XY-variant genetic disorder, especially as there are many myths out there about these children. However, parents are often confronted by the fact that their child may not have access to IEP services without disclosing the diagnosis.

o *"I understand your concerns about disclosure. My bigger concern is that without the services that he needs, he may not be successful. And to get him those services we need to disclose this. Let's discuss ways of talking to the school so we can assure you that the information will be confidential. For example, where will the school keep the records? Will kids or parents working in the office have access to these records? Let's talk about ways that the school can limit the number of people who will see this. Also, disclosing can help the school understand your child better. My guess is that the school might suspect there is something else going on. By giving the school that information—it might be an 'ah-ha' moment for them, 'Oh! Now it makes sense why he's not doing well.' More information can many times be better than less information."*

—*Jennifer Janusz, Psy.D.*

SICKLE CELL ANEMIA

Explaining sickle cell disease

Many families are not highly educated about the sickle cell disease process. Sometimes this is exacerbated by the fact that they are new immigrants with language barriers.

It's helpful to start off with a very basic explanation. They often view the disease as a hematological disorder. The idea that brains might be affected may be new to them.

○ *"I know that you've been told this is a blood disorder, and that's true. But our blood circulates through our entire body, including our brain. You know when your child has a crisis and it hurts them so badly? That's because the blood cells are blocking the vessel and not allowing the blood to go through properly and so the area that's next in line hurts because the blood didn't reach it. It's kind of the same in your brain. When the blood cells get blocked up because they are sickled, the blood doesn't reach the areas it should and those areas can be hurt or damaged. My job is to understand how this is affecting how your child thinks and learns."*

—*Laura Janzen, Ph.D.*

Explaining preventative interventions for sickle cell disease

With the sickle cell population, neuropsychologists almost always see clinical referrals when there has been positive neuroimaging (silent strokes), or school problems have already been recognized. With sickle cell, there is something that can be done. In this context, one important focus of the neuropsychological feedback is prevention.

○ *"We don't really know what will happen in the future. Disease management is so important. But some of this can be prevented in the future. For example, blood transfusions can prevent your child from having ongoing strokes. It's so important that you listen to what the team is suggesting. It can help your child feel better physically, but it can also help them avoid further strokes. So they can learn better and achieve better."*

—*Laura Janzen, Ph.D.*

Communicating with schools about sickle cell disease

The advocacy and liaison role for neuropsychologists is significant with sickle cell patients. Unlike the cancer population, typically there are no nurse specialists or school liaison social workers who can offer this communication. Within the feedback session, it is important to promote the idea that this assessment information is essential for the school in order to help with the child's learning; the same conversation needs to take place with the school team. The school staff are usually totally unaware of the issues. So the role of the neuropsychologist becomes one of educating the team as well as the family.

○ *I use handouts for teachers. This is a simple and effective strategy. I send multiple copies to the school. It covers topics like: "Do you know what the disease is? If a child misses a lot of school, how to plan for homework? The child may be tired and lethargic, but it's not because they are lazy; there are blood reasons why." The information is very basic.*

—*Laura Janzen, Ph.D.*

NEUROFIBROMATOSIS (NF)

Feedback with families of neurofibromatosis patients may involve addressing complex intergenerational issues. While it is well known to run in families, the accompanying lack of awareness of deficits can result in parents' not recognizing their own social or learning difficulties as being associated with NF until the feedback session for their child. Likewise, spouses might recognize for the first time what they now realize are NF traits in their husband or wife. Discussing the emotional consequences associated with visible plexiforms is also a topic frequently covered in feedback sessions.

Neurofibromatosis: When Discussing Shared Characteristics or Deficits in the Child and Parent

> o *"Mr. Smith, you have talked about how you had a hard time paying attention in school, related to your NF. These are the same kinds of things your child is going through."* (Even though we recognize that the parent may have cognitive issues related to NF, which can result in a lack of insight, it can still sometimes be surprising when the parent does not recognize similar traits in his/her child with the same disorder).
>
> —Jennifer Janusz, Psy.D.

Social/emotional consequences of facial plexiforms

Some kids have very disfiguring facial plexiforms. In these cases, it is important to speak with families regarding the social/emotional implications, in addition to the frequently significant learning issues.

> o *"There are a lot of aspects that put him at risk. He has a lot of learning problems, and he's a little socially awkward and that puts him at risk. But on top of this he also has a very visible tumor, and this is going to put him at greater risk socially. We can more easily intervene for the learning problems by getting his special education services and IEP in place. Unfortunately, we can't treat the facial tumor, but we can do things to help him socially. For example, how do we help him find things he is good at, keep him engaged with his small group of friends, and keep his self-esteem up, despite the risk factors that he has?"*
>
> —Jennifer Janusz, Psy.D.

SEIZURES AND EPILEPSY

The focus of the feedback session varies with the neuropsychologist's role in the seizure treatment team. Some neuropsychologists conduct assessments as part of a broader assessment of the patient's candidacy for neurosurgical resections, and may also be involved in Wada testing. In these cases, feedback sessions will include discussion of possible cognitive changes associated with the surgery. When seizures can be managed with medication, the focus of the feedback session is often a complex conversation regarding the origins of the day-to-day cognitive difficulties, including underlying lesions that are a common etiology for both seizure activity and cognitive deficits, medication effects, the impact of breakthrough seizure activity, and emotional issues.

Explaining the Impact of EEG Spikes

o *"You may have seen the EEG from the neurologist's report and noticed they talked about frequent 'spiking.' Your brain has a normal level of baseline activity. When they talk about these spikes, it's like a spark. Like you're trying to light a gas grill. And, most of the time those sparks are just that. There are sparks, and then everything goes back to normal. But every once in a while, those sparks will start a little kindling. And that's what you see when you see a seizure. But even when those sparks don't turn into a seizure, they can still affect how well Johnny concentrates, how he is able to listen to you, or how he remembers what he is doing in the middle of a task."*

—*Michael Westerveld, Ph.D.*

This is a way of explaining atypical EEGs and their effects on attention:

o *"There are little flashes going off in the brain. They aren't strong enough to be seizures, but they can disrupt attention."*

—*Molly Warner, Ph.D.*

Memory and Seizure Disorders

o *"People with epilepsy often have memory problems. First, you have the seizures themselves, and they dampen memory function. And then you have the treatment for the seizures—surgery can dampen memory function and so can the drugs. Finally, epilepsy is a tough disease to have, and depression that goes along with it can also affect memory. It's really a triple whammy to your memory function: the seizures, the treatment, and mood."*

—*Bill Barr, Ph.D.*

Attention and seizure disorders

Base rates of ADHD are about five to seven times greater in the epilepsy population than in general population. Often, they are both symptoms of something going on below.

o *"ADHD is very common in the epilepsy population, much more so than in general population. Often, the seizures and the inattention are both symptoms of something going on below, something that happened in John's brain. What happens clinically is that there are multiple factors affecting attention. The medication for seizures can affect attention. Then, those blips on the EEG, that interictal activity—that will cause inattention, and then of course the absence seizure—the behavioral manifestation will cause inattention."*

—*Bill MacAllister, Ph.D.*

House foundation metaphor for explaining the effect of loss of learning during critical periods

Parents frequently want to know (and hope) that if their child stops seizing today, they will be able to return to normal. Of course, the answer is often not as simple as this. For example, it depends on a number of issues, including the child's developmental course and when their course was altered by the neurological insult, as well as how much time has gone by and how much development has occurred. This can be explained to parents by using the metaphor of laying down the foundation for a house.

○ *"The foundation for this house was laid under adverse conditions. The foundation was laid during a storm. The ground was not solid, and now at this point, even if conditions are favorable, and you can build your house on top of this foundation without storms, without problems, still the foundation is not solid. It was not laid properly. So there are going to be limits on the future building on that site.*

"The foundation was already laid and it can't be redone. Especially when there's a period of time of really rapid early development, like in the first couple years of life, or even in the third and fourth year of life. You see enormous changes in children at this age, and of course it comes with substantial changes in the architecture of the brain. When your child learns something, there's a real live connection being made in the brain between neurons and centers of the brain that are now working together to become more sophisticated, to understand social interactions, maybe, or to comprehend language, and so on." (I try to describe the idea of a critical period without saying the phrase "critical period.") "If that period of time when there's rapid progress is disrupted, you don't get that period of time back. It's not like you can put that period of time on pause, and once conditions are more favorable un-pause it and start fresh. It doesn't work like that. It's not just like a time lag. There's been an opportunity that was not taken full advantage of, and there are ripple effects from that disruption. That disruption is not encapsulated in that period of time but carries through into later development.

So, even if your child stops having seizures today, we would still have some difficulties to talk about for him a couple of years from now. Would he make better developmental progress than he would otherwise? I would expect yes. But will the primary difficulties he has now go away? I would really guess no."
—*Katrina Boyer, Ph.D.*

Explaining the effect of untreated seizure disorders

○ *"It's like a repeated injury, and with repeated injuries come long-term consequences. And those long-term consequences result in some of the cells getting sick or dying. Over time, the cumulative effects are significant. It's like having one injury after another after another. If you break your arm three or four times, it just gets worse over time and it's harder to fix. With the first time, they put it together and works pretty well. You might be able to tell when the weather's going to change,*

*but it's okay. The second time, it's harder to put it back together, and by the third
or fourth time you can expect to become less and less functional each time."*

—*Jim Scott, Ph.D.*

Explaining the impact of subclinical seizures

When a seizure disorder is associated with a childhood encephalopathy that has frequent nocturnal discharges, it can be challenging for parents to understand why their child needs medication, especially if there are no, or very few, obvious seizures that occur during the day. In relatively rare situations where the neurologist suspect an epilepsy syndrome involving epileptic encephalopathy, I will help the family understand how this neurological phenomenon may affect their child's development.

> o *"Your child has frequent epileptic discharges in between seizures, especially in sleep. You're aware of this"* (check in with parents to be clear that the neurologist has described the concept of epileptic encephalopathy to them). *"It's not necessarily the number of seizures the person has, but this level of activity that is below the surface—the seizures are like the tip of the iceberg, and what you don't see underwater, that's still the iceberg. There's all this underneath the surface that's not erupting into a seizure that's problematic, and in certain cases that abnormal activity is mostly seen during sleep."* (I'll talk about why that is particularly disruptive to learning and memory and development in general.) *"All the things your child does during the day to make associations between concepts, to learn new words, to engage in new experiences—all of that is a very active level of processing. And when the child goes to sleep, the child is more passive; however, the brain actually becomes very active in consolidating experiences and information that's been gathered in the day. Connections between these experiences and past experiences are made, and that consolidation happens during sleep. If the child is having abnormal epileptic discharges and that period of sleep is disrupted, information may not become consolidated as well. If this occurs night after night, it takes a toll on that person's development of new concepts, their learning, their memory in general. Hypothetically speaking, it may alter how efficiently that person's thinking networks are established. So even if your child isn't having a seizure that you can see, we believe this activity is problematic for their learning, memory, and general development over time."*

—*Katrina Boyer, Ph.D.*

Seizure medications and cognitive functioning

Seizure medications can cause sedation and inattention. It's important to stress both the side effects and the benefits of the medication as a package: uncontrolled seizures can be dangerous, and one does not want to give parents or patients the notion that the origin of the attention or memory problem is the seizure medications, as opposed to the seizures, which cause the need to have seizures medications in the first place. At the same time, if assessment reveals substantial attention deficits, suggesting a discussion with the prescribing clinician may result in an appropriate titration of medication and relief for some of these difficulties. Careful wording and checking in with families to ensure that they understand the complexities of the situation is highly recommended.

o *"Uncontrolled seizures can be very harmful, especially if they become long. That can be very dangerous and harmful. Still, I observed that James seemed very sedated after he took his antiseizure medication. You may want to go back and inquire if there is a different medication regime that will make your child less sedated."*
   —*Laura Janzen, Ph.D.*

o *"The memory problems that go along with taking seizure medications are really a 'Catch-22.' If you give these medications to people without seizures, they report memory problems. So we know that, independent of the seizures, these medications can dampen memory function. But, and here's the Catch-22, if you have seizures, and you don't take the medications, your memory function is much worse because of the increase in seizure activity. So our goal is to treat the seizures as effectively as possible with as few drugs as possible."*
   —*Bill Barr, Ph.D.*

Often parents will come in and say that before their child started this medication, they were "fine" (or at least better) and then things got worse. I try to help them understand their child's story a little better. I walk them through the logic of their explanation and what other possible explanations there may be: they start having seizures, they start a medication, years go by, and now things are worse. If we just remove the medication, will things really be better for this kid? Yes, it's possible.

o *"But ... if that medication has had adverse effects, those adverse effects have been in play for a period of your child's development. Just lifting that medication doesn't change the impact that has already been made by that medication over time. Then you have to factor in, not only did your child have that medication, but the reason for the medication is this epilepsy syndrome and that's been co-occurring with the medication, and of course, is very likely part of the problem."*

   A lot of times parents want to believe it's the medication that is making the child worse and that it's nothing specific to their child. They don't want their child to be damaged; they want it to be the drugs.
   —*Katrina Boyer, Ph.D.*

Explaining the need for seizure medications

This is the one time where I might cite the literature about percentages. A lot of families go on the Internet and read really frightening information about anti-epileptic medications. This tells you that they have a thirst for information and they want to understand.

o *"Just like everything else—they can say this medication is safe for 90 to 95 percent of people. But five percent might have a reaction, maybe your child is one of those five. And no one knows how to predict if your child will be one of those kids who has trouble concentrating because of the medication, not because of the seizures. But a much worse alternative is just letting him have the seizures."*
—*Michael Westerveld, Ph.D.*

Normalizing Mood Issues in Epilepsy

o *"I don't know everything about your life. Everyone has things to be depressed about. But you also have this condition. Of course you would rather be doing other things than dealing with seizures. It's common to have some depression around this."*
—*Bill Barr, Ph.D.*

NONEPILEPTIC SEIZURES/PSEUDOSEIZURES

Some patients have electrographic correlates to their seizures, and some do not. As the literature shows, some patients may experience "real" seizures in addition to pseudoseizures. Explaining to a person that they are not having the type of seizure that has an EEG correlate is a delicate process, and one that can be enhanced further through the pearls below as well as through a review of Chapter 8 "Somatoform Disorders."

Explaining pseudoseizures to patients without losing rapport

If you just say, "Those aren't seizures" and that's the patient's identity—it's fulfilling some kind of need for them—you have stripped some of their identity from them. They will just argue with you that they are experiencing "spells," and feel like you've missed something. You're a "bad doctor." You have to approach this conversation carefully.

o *"There are different types of seizures and different causes for seizures or spells. Some have electrographic correlates, and some don't. You're lucky, you have the kind that are not associated with electrical abnormalities in your brain. And that makes them more treatable. This is really good news. There's different ways these types of seizures are treated and they can be completely treated. Sometimes we have things that we are trying to cope with emotionally that are difficult and we're not really able to bring that out and cope with it. And it comes out this way. In these spells— these are real. These are real spells you're having. And they can be treated with psychotherapy and counseling."*
—*Sara J. Swanson, Ph.D.*

Patients can often tell the difference between pseudoseizures and ones with EEG correlates: "Oh yeah—those are my little spells and my big spells." I never use the term "fake."

o "*You have some seizures that are what we would call 'real,' and others that seem to come from stress or other things. Let's talk about what we saw on the monitoring. These are spells without any abnormalities on our lab tests*" (as opposed to spells with abnormalities on the lab tests). "*What are some of the ways you control them?*"

—*Roberta F. White, Ph.D.*

EPILEPSY SURGERY

During a consent procedure with neurosurgeons, families will sometimes leave without a full understanding of the issues surrounding the surgery. The neuropsychological feedback session is another opportunity to help them develop a more comprehensive appreciation of the potential risks and advantages of the upcoming procedure. Feedback sessions that occur following surgery can also be a means to help explain any loss of cognitive function, or paradoxically, loss of disability.

Bad Brain Is Worse Than No Brain Metaphor for Epilepsy Surgery Consideration

o "*Well, you know 'bad brain is worse than no brain,' because the seizure focus in the brain is not working to begin with, and it's interfering with the rest of the brain's ability to do its work. Now, sometimes as part of the surgery, because it's imprecise or hard to identify exactly where the bad cells end and the good cells start, you might see some changes in the functioning of the 'good brain' after surgery. Those changes might take a while to normalize. In the first few months after surgery, you may see*" (X and Y), "*and in the next several months, you will see*" (A and B). "*At a certain point, more normal development for your child will take place. The transition will take place due to healing from the surgery, and due to resuming a more normal trajectory of development. If she doesn't have the surgery, sometimes the surgeon is concerned that the development is going to be constantly interrupted.*"

—*Michael Westerveld, Ph.D.*

Epilepsy Surgery Consideration—What Are Your Goals?

o "*You need to understand the potential. He might take a long time to wake up after surgery. He may also drop a few IQ points. Those points might make the difference between him being able to live independently* [or not]. *Let's talk about the potential downsides here.*"

—*Marc Norman, Ph.D.*

Memory and Epilepsy Surgery

o "*If we take out that left temporal lobe, your child will lose memory skills. But in 10 years, because of the effects of uncontrolled seizures, he won't have that memory*

*anyway. So" (paraphrasing my colleague, Bill Barr) "the question is, do you want
your child to live seizure-free for the next 10 years and take the memory hit now,
or have seizures for the next 10 years, and eventually get the memory problem? You
can expect that four months after surgery, the IQ goes down, but then a year later,
it is better than when they started. It's a rocky road in the beginning, but at the
end of the tunnel they will be better off."*

—*Bill MacAllister, Ph.D.*

Acute recovery expectations following epilepsy surgery

Feedback sessions with epilepsy patients destined for surgical treatment are a good
opportunity to forewarn patients and families about some common post-surgical
neurological symptoms, *prior* to their epilepsy surgery. This practice can make the
recovery phase significantly less stressful. If and when symptoms emerge in the acute
post-surgical phase, they are expected, as opposed to a nightmarish surprise that elicits fears like, "They slipped! I'm going to be damaged for life!"

   o *"Listen, when you wake up from surgery, you will probably have some major neurological symptoms. You might not be able to speak or move things. A lot of things
   could be going on. Ninety percent or more of these types of symptoms will be temporary and will resolve over a period of days to weeks—months on the outside. So
   don't be surprised or freaked out if you can't (a, b, or c). Because there is a lot of
   swelling—surgery is a major traumatic event—the brain can take a while to sort
   it all out."*

—*Aaron Nelson, Ph.D.*

Successful epilepsy surgery—what now?

Successful epilepsy surgery can paradoxically create a loss. Many patients comment, "It's like losing my best friend." From the patient's perspective, the feedback session is just not about scores, it's about a huge psychological shift into
the world of healthy people. Some have unrealistic expectations that need to be
addressed. For these patients, the feedback session is more like a vocational counseling session.

   o *"So, what does this all mean for you in terms of entering the healthy population?
   The question we need to address is 'What now?'"*

—*Gordon Chelune, Ph.D.*

PREMATURITY

Something to Consider: It's important to keep in mind the psychosocial stressors
families of preemies have been through well before they get to you. Usually when
the baby is born, they don't know what is happening. They are unprepared psycho-
logically for the baby, and the practical aspects can be overwhelming. How does one

spend three months in the NICU?! And the baby is very fragile. As a neuropsychologist working with the family later on in the child's life, you don't know what the parents were told when he or she was born "We don't know whether she will live … your child will have all kinds of problems.… " Spending all that time in the NICU does a lot to families. Their reaction is often not something they talk about, but it contributes to an underlying theme that drives their perspective. The fact that they can't take their baby home and bond in the typical way—parents carry a guilt about that, especially the mothers. That's understandable, but usually not factual. This guilt often drives their interactions with the providers. The other thing is that they have this whole process where they worry the baby won't live, and then when they make it through that horrific period, they are then told, "You'll just have to deal with some subtle learning problems." "Oh, is that all!? I can live with that."

But maybe when the child turns six or seven, the learning issues are not so subtle. Over the course of their child's (short) lifetime, parents can be given a lot of confusing and conflicting information about what to expect for the child. That and the guilt are the backdrops for these families. Helping them come to grips with the idea that this is something that they will be dealing with over the long haul and that the challenges will change over time is an important goal when working with these families. One of the most comforting things is to put the pieces together; give them knowledge. They may have seen a number of providers who gave them a piece of information, but no one has put it together. I try to understand what a parent has understood from prior provider consultations:

"What was the conclusion that came from the neurologist visits?" (Often they don't get the big picture; e.g., they may not realize their child's brain has been damaged). I try to make sure they understand what they are dealing with (e.g., with stroke or hydrocephalus). I may say explicitly, "Your child had some neurological damage."

—E. Mark Mahone, Ph.D.

HYDROCEPHALUS

One goal of feedback sessions for patients with hydrocephalus is to ensure a basic understanding of the mechanisms of hydrocephalus and shunt placement. Counseling patients and their families about red-flag symptoms that should trigger concern about shunt failure is also important.

Clogged Drain Metaphor for Hydrocephalus

o *I have a picture of ventricular system that I refer to during this conversation: "When the drains get clogged, the ventricles swell up and you get hydrocephalus. When your child has a shunt, in theory, things should be stable. But in practice, it doesn't always happen that way. Kids can have variable cognitive profiles, day to day, and morning to afternoon, as a result of variability of intracranial pressure. And even though the shunts are pretty good, the reality is that you need to be on the lookout for signs that might reflect shunt malfunction. We will cross our fingers, and hope it works well. But it's important to be prepared."*

—E. Mark Mahone, Ph.D.

Overinflated Balloon Metaphor for the Impact of Hydrocephalus on the Ventricles

○ *"If you take a balloon and keep blowing it up, eventually the latex gets distended so it doesn't pop back into shape as well when you deflate it. That potentially happens with some of the white matter around the ventricles. If it continues to get pulled and sheared, even when the ventricle size is back to normal, the white matter tracks around the ventricles may be still stretched out, and that can become a problem."*

—E. Mark Mahone, Ph.D.

Explaining Why a Child Needs a Shunt

○ *"The reason that this child needs the shunt, is that this structure"* (point to head), *"called the cerebellum, is not in the right spot. It blocks the circulation of fluid through the central nervous system, and that's why we needed the shunt in the first place. The cerebellum is important for motor planning and balance. And on top of that your son also has a spinal cord lesion—he can't feel or control anything below that lesion. Those two things together make walking difficult.*

"A lot of kids with cerebellum problems and shunts also have trouble with executive functioning skills. Even when IQ is average or low average, they can have trouble with problem solving and reaching their goals. Up until around 15 years ago, we thought the cerebellum was just for motor skills. But now we know this area is important for problem solving and pulling together information. We know he will be at risk for these types of issues as well. In addition, having the shunt means that at some point the pressure in his brain was higher. That's why the shunt was placed—to prevent that from happening again. However, shunt malfunctions and infections can cause the pressure can go up, which can further affect his thinking abilities."

—Jennifer Turek Queally, Ph.D.

SPINA BIFIDA

Spina bifida develops during the first month of a child's gestational development (i.e., during the first month of pregnancy). With currently available imaging technology, this means that parents have generally made a conscious choice to bring their child into the world despite knowing about his or her condition. This can create very complicated layers of emotional reactions in the context of feedback sessions.

o *"There is nothing about this condition that you are prepared to deal with as a parent. It's atypical, so we have to adopt an atypical approach. When you are supposed to be separating during your teenage years, the level of dependence upon parents can actually be intensifying."*

—Andrew Zabel, Ph.D.

Because many obstetrical practices encourage abortion, when parents recognize the full effect of the decision to bring their child into the world, with a full sense of what they will go through, the reaction can be very emotionally complicated. Sometimes parents will be defensive (e.g., "my child has no shunt—so there won't be any learning issues"). This can be further magnified when their child has developed relatively strong language skills.

o *"Let's think about his early development, and how it was different. When he had problems moving, he didn't crawl under the coffee table to try to get things out. He didn't work on spatial relationships in the same way—'how fast does my body go, where does it fit?' Instead he is in one place, using his language: 'Mom! Come play! Mom, bring me this! Mom! Look what I can do!' You probably saw early that his language skills were better developed than his spatial skills.*

"And we see that over time—that profile stays in place. He started working on those skills earlier. They stayed stronger. And because they are stronger he tends to rely on them more heavily when he does visual-spatial or visual-motor skills. So now, 10 years later, we see a big difference between the two skill sets."

—Jennifer Turek Queally, Ph.D.

CEREBRAL PALSY (CP)

Something to consider: Some parents who have children with CP overestimate their child's cognitive capabilities, and attribute much of their functional limitations to physical impairments. This belief can limit the family's ability to take advantage of interventions that the child may really need.

I suspect that many families hold desperately to the "locked in" scenario because they lack an optimistic alternative. If they abandon the idea of entirely normal cognition in their child, they don't have anything. I think it is our job to help them establish a new vision for their child's education and skill development without crushing the deeper vision of their child having a meaningful and happy life. This involves a refinement of the belief system, not a refutation. You will not be able to pull the carpet out from under them and get them to accept their child's cognitive delays or limitations. You need to refocus the vision, and help the family hang their hat on a new possibility and a goal state that is entirely possible despite the cognitive limitations. You have to give them something else to believe in.

—Andrew Zabel, Ph.D.

MULTIPLE SCLEROSIS (MS)

Initial neuropsychological feedback sessions with MS patients may occur prior to their diagnosis; cognitive test findings tend to be only one piece of what is typically a complex puzzle that can take months or years to assemble. In these instances, feedback may not involve a discussion of the diagnosis per se, although certainly a patient's cognitive deficits and their impact on day-to-day functioning should be explored. Nonetheless, sometimes this feedback session may involve a discussion of MS in general, to help patients better understand the condition that is being considered as a primary differential diagnosis. Feedback with patients who have a well-established MS diagnosis may emphasize the effects of cognitive changes on a patient's ability to function at work and home, and compensatory strategies to maintain function. It may also address a patient's lack of awareness of cognitive deficits and personality changes, as well as the effects of mood on functioning.

Explaining MS and the Brain

○ *"There are these special fibers in the brain that carry messages over relatively long distances, and they are covered by these special insulating sheaths. That allows the messages to be carried even faster, and enable the communication at high speed across the brain. In MS those fibers are damaged."*

—Robert H. Bilder, Ph.D.

Helping patients explain their deficits to others despite their healthy appearance

MS patients often look well from the outside, and are puzzled about why their interactions with co-workers or spouses aren't going well. They might have trouble with deficits one afternoon when they are tired, only to look better the next morning. One goal is to help MS patients appreciate why others may not understand them. I like to introduce the concept that others might perceive you incorrectly because of the nature of MS, and that the patient has the ability to help correct this.

○ *"Others might perceive you incorrectly. These tests show you have some difficulty with processing information quickly and retrieving information. But people might not appreciate from the outside your fatigue or mental slowing. Or they may not realize that you can do a task in the morning and have a lot of trouble with that same task in the afternoon."* (In these cases I will recommend that the patient see if there is a way that he can ask his employer to split his time, or to take a longer lunch break.)

—Gordon Chelune, Ph.D.

Encouraging the need for self-care in patients with ms

Some patients have a stiff-upper-lip approach, "By God, I'm not going to let this affect me...." I recall one patient who was financially burdened. So she didn't quit her second job, and sleep deprivation was interfering with her cognition.

o *"Here's your prescription: you need to get at least eight hours' sleep per night. I know it's going to be difficult, but you need to do this. I want to see you back in a month, and I want to hear your plan."*

—*Gordon Chelune, Ph.D.*

Limits of Assessment in MS

o *Sometimes you write things in reports and they come back to bite you (e.g., patients may be denied disability even when their condition warrants it). This can be especially important when patients have MS, as their limiting symptoms may not be measured by cognitive tests. So, I often add a line in my report to acknowledge this: "Neuropsychological testing does not produce valid information about fatigue, pain, and other MS symptoms that might impact work capacity."*

—*Margaret O'Connor, Ph.D.*

HEPATITIS

Research shows that interferon can increase impulsivity. This is one way of explaining the increased risks of interferon use when there is a previous history of impulsive behavior.

o *"Everything in medicine is a risk–benefit ratio. Everything has side effects. The physician always has to evaluate the benefits and risks. If the risk outweighs the benefit, then it won't be helpful. This medicine can make things bubble to the surface. It can also help with the hepatitis. So, here's the dilemma, 'If I take interferon, I can add 10 years to my life, but there is a risk that I could kill myself.' If there are issues in the past or propensities for self-harm, depression, suicidal ideation, it has a tendency to bubble that to the surface, even if you are doing well now."*

—*Robert (Bob) Denney, Psy.D.*

HUMAN IMMUNODEFICIENCY VIRUS

Prior to the neuropsychological encounter, some patients with HIV may have been told they have dementia. However, the term "AIDS or HIV dementia" may not be helpful because of the incorrect assumptions patients may make about their anticipated course of cognitive changes. This misinformation often needs to be corrected as part of the feedback process. More generally, when giving feedback to patients with HIV and AIDS, other issues involving basic health and safety such as whether their families know their status, medication compliance, and substance abuse issues also need to be addressed.

HIV's Effect on the Brain

o *"You've heard a great deal about how HIV affects the body. That's what we all hear about; how it can cause problems with cancer and other things. What we*

don't talk a lot about is its impact on the brain. Did you know HIV can affect the
brain? It's important that you know about that—that this is something that can
happen—so you can talk to your doctor about this."

—Monica Mindt, Ph.D.

o "Just because you have problems now, doesn't mean you will always have problems.
Or that it will get worse. It's important for you to come back so we can continue taking a look at this. You can talk to your doctor … and maybe there are some things
you can do to function better" (insert talk about taking medications regularly here).

—Monica Mindt, Ph.D.

HIV Dementia

o "Unlike other forms of dementia, like Alzheimer disease, this dementia isn't
necessarily progressive. It is affected by compliance. Since HIV crosses into
the brain, your best defense is to take good care of yourself. Take your HIV
medication."

—Desirée White, Ph.D.

Substance abuse and HIV

Bringing up treatment for substance abuse without pushing it is delicate. One technique is to orient the discussion around questions. When you approach things from
the perspective of a question, people are less likely to feel judged.

o "I see that you're not doing well. You're having these problems that you were not
having before. And you mentioned that you aren't able to take your medicines
regularly. And you said you were still using. I wonder if you think that there is a
connection? Do you think using is impacting taking your meds?"

—Monica Mindt, Ph.D.

Other times, it makes sense to take a more direct approach:

o "Okay, when you're using—how can you also continue taking your meds?"

—Monica Mindt, Ph.D.

Addressing the full range of needs in patients with hiv

Something to consider: When working with HIV populations, feedback sessions
often go well beyond discussing test scores. The feedback is an opportunity to affect
the patient's overall health and discuss basic services. Clinicians can review with
patients where they can stay if they do not have housing, and where they can access
food.

—Monica Mindt, Ph.D.

Some patients live with families that don't know their HIV status. They keep their medications in a closet in the back room—and they can't easily get to them. There might even be safety concerns if their status is disclosed. Feedback sessions involve lots of listening, and not being judgmental; respecting a client's values and the values of their family. Based on THEIR reality—this is where they're going back, how can we make this better? If a clinician didn't know better, they would just say something like, "You should take you meds regularly," and they (the patient) would say "okay." This would be a huge opportunity lost for really figuring out how to help them.

o *"I think it would really help if you could take your medicines more regularly. And I wonder if we could problem-solve about a safety plan so you can do that."*

—*Monica Mindt, Ph.D.*

14 Addressing Effort

OVER THE PAST decade, our field's capacity to detect patients' suboptimal effort has expanded in conjunction with an appreciation for the need of such assessment procedures. For example, the American Academy of Clinical Neuropsychology Consensus Conference Statement on the Neuropsychological Assessment of Effort, Response Bias, and Malingering (Heilbronner et al., 2010) highlights that while the base rate of suboptimal effort is higher in litigating or forensic settings, response bias occurs in routine medical and clinical settings as well. Consequently, the consensus statement includes a recommendation for the routine use of both standalone and embedded symptom validity measures even in clinical practice without any forensic involvement.

As the routine assessment of response bias is more actively incorporated into daily practice, many clinicians find that constructive communication of suboptimal effort to patients is as much, or more of a clinical challenge as response bias detection itself. While the response bias literature has expanded in the past decade, the literature on clinical communication of response bias remains nascent. Carone, Iverson, and Bush (2010) point out that this gap is due in part to the fact that the development of symptom validity testing has primarily emerged in the forensic setting where the nature of the neuropsychologist–examinee relationship typically precludes feedback.

This chapter includes strategies to address effort with patients. Clinicians we spoke with stressed their intentions to use effort data to open up a productive dialogue with patients during *clinical* assessments. Their approaches may differ when completing a forensic based evaluation, as the goals of such assessments are often quite different.

TIMING OF FEEDBACK REGARDING SUBOPTIMAL EFFORT

Depending on the reason for referral (i.e., clinical versus forensic), some clinicians provide feedback about poor effort as soon as a symptom validity test is failed in the course of testing. Those who provide immediate feedback often do so in the hope that patients will respond with greater effort, particularly in medical settings where scant resources preclude repeat evaluations on later dates, or the timing of upcoming surgical decisions depends on eliciting the best possible performance from patients during the current assessment.

Clinicians likewise vary in their willingness to continue testing once effort issues have been uncovered. Some discontinue testing immediately; others continue with the assessment, typically with the goal of gathering convergent data on effort. Another benefit of continued assessment is the ability to report at least minimal levels of functioning in cognitive domains. That is, despite suboptimal effort, cognitive testing may demonstrate at least average language function, or at least average intellect.

Addressing suboptimal effort with patients during the assessment

o *"Wow! You just failed a test that even patients with Alzheimer's can do. Why is that? If you keep doing this, I won't be able to interpret your neuropsychological tests."*

—*Roberta F. White, Ph.D.*

Addressing trust with patients who fail symptom validity tests

Failure on a symptom validity test can be an opportunity to see what need is being fulfilled. Sometimes, patients feel no one believes them, and therefore exaggerate on the tests. In this case, a patient was seen five years previously, after a well-documented severe TBI with coma, while he was still in the acute stage. He failed the symptom validity tests on the current evaluation. This issue can be framed, not as "Are you trying or not trying?" but rather, "Are you going to trust me?"

o *"Well, I know you had a significant head injury. So significant I am convinced you have documentable residua. You are just trying to prove it too hard. Look, you have to trust me. I really need you to do your best."*

—*Roberta F. White, Ph.D.*

Reassuring Patients of Test Sensitivity

o *"For some reason, you're not being able to put forth your best effort on some of these tests, and I don't know why that is." (Or, more forcefully, "These results aren't making sense. There are inconsistencies. Some of your results are far worse than for people with Alzheimer disease.") "I need you to try your best. These tests are sensitive; you don't need to exaggerate the problems you think you are having in order to show us."*

—*Munro Cullum, Ph.D.*

Addressing effort with pre-surgical patients

When pre-surgical patients fail symptom validity tests, neuropsychologists are faced with a difficult situation. In other domains of practice, they might not allow patients to retake tests, assuming that data are suspect once poor effort has been detected. However, particularly on multidisciplinary teams, the question becomes, "Dr. Smith, why didn't you get good effort?" One strategy is to clearly address the poor effort in the feedback session and then invite the patient to return to retake the tests.

o *"I know you were trying in many areas. But these test results suggest that in some areas you had a hard time applying yourself or keeping motivated. You can come back to re-do the tests, but you will really have to apply yourself."*

—*Bill Barr, Ph.D.*

As with providing feedback on any clinical phenomenon, social pragmatics and careful language choice are important when engaging and educating patients about the nature and impact of their effort on neuropsychological assessment results. Use of words like "malingering" or "faking" may be inaccurate in the context of a continuum of effort (e.g., Heilbronner et al., 2010). This concept of a continuum recognizes that effort may vary over the course of an evaluation, and that poor effort might span a range of behaviors: from lack of exertion on a task through exerting effort to appear impaired. Carone et. al. (2010) suggest that even when accurate, use of words like "poor effort" or "faking" is too emotionally loaded. They are more constructively replaced with "not fully invested" or "disengaged." If the feedback feels like an accusation, patients are more likely to respond defensively. The following are strategies to open up a productive dialogue.

Disengaged metaphor for effort

The terminology one uses with patients is important. If you say to a patient who fails effort testing, "Did you try your best?" they will almost always tell you, "Yes." If you use terms like "disengage," they may admit that they were not fully engaged because it sounds less like cheating. The term *disengaged* is not sugarcoating it. In the report, clinicians can then document, "We discussed, and patient acknowledged, that there are times when he disengaged during the evaluation."

> o *"Well, you know what, I'm looking over this testing. There's something that suggests to me that you tend to get overwhelmed at times when you're stressed. When that happens you disengage from what you're doing. What do you think about that? Do you think that's something that you might do?" "Yes! That's exactly what happens sometimes."*
> — Dominic Carone, Ph.D.

After introducing the concept of disengagement, it helps to show patients a graph of test results.

> o *"Will you agree that you are smarter than someone who had the diagnosis of mental retardation?" ("Yes.") "Well, I agree with you. Okay, so look. Here's a test I gave you. Now look, you have mild injury. Here's this group of mentally retarded adults. Here's moderate to severe TBI patients: you are way down here. That doesn't make sense. Neurologically, I'm kind of scratching my head.... Do you know of any medical condition where the patient who has the lesser/milder condition will report more symptoms than the severe version of the disease ... for example, with heart disease? There is something going on here with this disengagement that is not neurological."*
> —Dominic Carone, Ph.D.

I see feedback with poor effort as a progression from: Do you see yourself as disengaging ... then your problems are not neurologically based ... then good news. The key is to come across as patient/client-centered. It is also important, though, not to use language that obfuscates. I don't say, "cry for help" when there is no evidence that they are seeking psychological help.

> o *"The good news is ... I have patients who I have to give really bad news. I don't have anything I can do for them to help them get better. In your case I think there's really good news. I don't think there's anything going on that's not controllable— that you have a brain injury you can't control. In your case, look at all these psychological symptoms. You're having anxiety attacks. You're going to the physician, OT, PT. In all these months, no one has ever sent you to a psychologist who can really help with these symptoms. Great news!"*
> —Dominic Carone, Ph.D.

Reframing poor effort as a clinical opportunity to understand patients

People not trying their best or manufacturing symptoms don't bother me, even though many clinicians can be angered by it. For me, if I can help the patient figure out what need the symptoms are addressing—it helps make the feedback session effective.

o *"Help me understand what's going on here. What do you think happened?"*
—Roberta F. White, Ph.D.

o *"You seem like a smart person. I know that you had this level of education, and you functioned at a high level. So when I get these test results, this is very confusing to me. There are some difficulties with these numbers, because most of the time, someone in your situation would score much higher." (Some people will say, "What if I was really anxious, or didn't get sleep?") "Well, those are things that can have some impact, but typically the impact of those factors on the test scores is something much less than that." (If there is some dissimulation....) "I don't see these kinds of scores except for people who have the most serious kind of neurological diseases, like Alzheimer disease. And I am pretty sure you don't have Alzheimer's. This is confusing—it's a difficult thing to figure out."*
—Greg Lamberty, Ph.D.

X-ray Metaphor for Effort

o *"Do you know how when you get an X-ray, or a CT scan, the technician tells you, 'Hold still! Don't move!' because if you move, the picture comes out fuzzy? It's impossible to read the X-ray picture because the movement has created 'static' that made everything blurred. It's the same thing with our assessments. You need to put forth your best effort, or the data is blurry and impossible to read. It's impossible to tell what your strengths and weaknesses are, and what is 'static.' Nothing makes sense. That's what happened with this assessment. I can't answer the question you brought here, because of the problem with effort."*
—Karen Postal, Ph.D.

LEARNING DISABILITY POPULATIONS

Many high school and college students are significantly motivated to be diagnosed with ADHD or other learning disabilities in order to gain accommodations such as extended time on the SAT or LSAT, access to services, and/or medications. As with litigation populations, some individuals with genuine ADHD will try to "demonstrate" the extent of their problems by exaggerating on tests. Others may be fabricating symptoms altogether, which has increased the need to incorporate effort testing when evaluating adolescents and young adults for the presence of these conditions. Similarly, clinicians are increasingly incorporating symptom validity tests and embedded validity measures in the context of child assessment. Effort testing with younger children brings its own unique constellation of difficulties, especially as a lack of "effort" in this population does not necessarily mean the child is attempting to "fake bad." For example, younger children may not have any perceived stake in the outcome of the assessment, and simply put forth no effort.

Driving analogy for sub-optimal effort

Unlike in medico-legal situations, many clinicians working with learning disability/ ADHD populations will give patients the benefit of the doubt and allow them to take tests again if effort looked bad. The following approach is particularly effective, because no teenager wants to be barred from driving.

> o *"For whatever reason, I don't think you gave your best effort. If you are this poor at paying attention, you shouldn't be driving. You're going to come back, and do it again, but this time you need to put everything into it."*
> —*Robb Mapou, Ph.D.*

Symptom Validity Tests (SVTs)

Children will occasionally fail symptom validity tests. I have struggled with how to give feedback to parents and kids in this situation. Do you give the feedback to everyone together? Do you stop testing right away? Do you wait, put all of the information together, and then give feedback? My general approach has been to continue with the evaluation, but to modify the test battery to some extent to allow for more time to explore the potential reasons the child is failing the SVTs. Obviously, you can fail a single effort test for multiple reasons. The clinician needs to determine whether this is an overall invalid protocol and what data are meaningful with regard to brain–behavior relationships and clinical management.

> o *"John was not consistently motivated to perform well. He had a hard time staying invested in the testing, in a way that is not typical for children of his age. I don't think his effort was consistently optimal across the testing session. Why do you think that is? Can you help me understand what might have happened?" (The next step depends on the particular circumstances. For example, if the patient's suboptimal effort was judged related to his difficulty at school …) "I thought John was really trying to show me that he is struggling at school and he wants more help."*
> —*Michael Kirkwood, Ph.D.*

REFERENCES

Carone DA, Iverson GL, Bush SS. [Image omitted] A model to approaching and providing feedback to patients regarding invalid test performance in clinical neuropsychological evaluations. *Clin Neuropsychol.* 2010;24(5):759–778.

Heilbronner et. al. The American Academy of Clinical Neuropsychology Consensus Conference Statement on the Neuropsychological Assessment of Effort, Response Bias, and Malingering. *Clin Neuropsychol.* 2010:23:7:1093–1129

III Communication Beyond the Feedback Session

15 Communicating Assessment Results to Other Professionals

COMMUNICATING NEUROPSYCHOLOGICAL assessment results to other professions takes place through a combination of written reports, interdisciplinary team meetings, and telephone calls. At medical centers and integrated group practices, it might also be possible to stop by the office of a colleague to share more informal feedback. Regardless of the communication method that we employ, being able to effectively provide feedback to referral sources and other treating professionals not only improves patient care, it supports a thriving practice. Keeping communication short, clearly outlining aspects of the referral question that could not be answered, and tailoring messages to referrers' areas of concern are common denominators in effective feedback strategies with professionals.

INTERDISCIPLINARY TEAMS

When neuropsychologists participate in interdisciplinary team meetings, clear, concise communication is critical. Members of the team from other disciplines are almost never interested in the minutiae of specific scores; they are seeking big-picture input that is grounded in real-world functioning. Is the patient demented? Is a mood disorder present, and if so, how will it affect the team's goals? Being scientifically sound and readily acknowledging when you don't have information is also critical. Experienced team members will say, "Let me get you that information," rather than hedge.

> When communicating results to other professionals, it's important to contextualize the neuropsychological data. The patient might have been referred from an interdisciplinary Parkinson's neurosurgery team. So, you want to clearly address the presumed question: are your results typical for Parkinson's? Rather than just saying "he has executive dysfunction," the data is most helpfully presented as being consistent with or inconsistent with the disease being addressed by the referral source.
>
> o *"What we are seeing here is very atypical for Parkinson disease"* (or name the disease process).
>> —*Cynthia Kubu, Ph.D.*

> Often, teams of professionals have to be reminded that cognitive dysfunction falls along a continuum. The patient may not be frankly demented, but may have significant cognitive impairments that the team should consider. For example, when working with an individual who is impulsive or hypersexual, a deep brain stimulator might improve motor control, but what would the behavioral outcome be?
>
> o *"This gentleman is on the slippery slope towards dementia. He has problems with reasoning and impulsivity and cannot live alone...."*
>> —*Cynthia Kubu Ph.D.*

Being the voice of the patient and family

Something to think about: Neuropsychologists often have the luxury of time that most other providers do not. We have the opportunity to interview family members and patients at length, which allows the neuropsychologist to become the voice of the family at interdisciplinary team meetings. For example, one can bring up non-motor issues that the team does not know about, and might affect quality of life, like hypersexuality, lack of hygiene, or mood issues.

> o *"During our assessment, the family indicated they are concerned about..."*
> —*Cynthia Kubu, Ph.D.*

GENERAL STRATEGIES FOR COMMUNICATING WITH OTHER PROFESSIONALS

When communicating results to other professionals, it is important to titrate what you are saying. Similar to our interactions with patients and their families, the first question to consider is often, "What are you most concerned about? What issues are you and/or the patient having the most difficulty with? What has been tried already that has worked, and has not worked?" Listening first creates the context of a productive dialogue about the patient.

When physician colleagues don't understand standard scores or other conclusions, they may respond with challenges, rather than questions. This is helpful to keep in mind, because a good response to "How could you say that!?" is not to get defensive, and to explain clearly what the scores mean. For example:

> o *"Mr. Smith scored at the 30th percentile; that's within the average range. So compared to the typical person his age, his memory is right on track."*
> —*Gordon Chelune, Ph.D.*

Speaking to other professionals through patients

Something to think about: It is important to keep in mind that, when you are speaking with patients, you are in a way speaking through them to other professionals. You can be certain that when they are done with you, they will go to the next doctor—and that doctor will say, oh, so what did Dr. Janzen tell you? It's important to be very thoughtful about those relationships.

> o *Imagine that the referring physician is sitting in the office hearing the results. If there is anything that you feel might feel undermining to her/him, rephrase it.*
> —*Laura Janzen, Ph.D.*

FEEDBACK TO IEP TEAMS

Many clinicians accompany families to IEP meetings or participate in such meetings by phone. During these meetings, neuropsychologists might feel that they are walking into hostile territory, or conversely, they may enjoy a collegial relationship with a well-known team. Over time, developing relationships with educational professionals helps clinicians become more effective in securing services for patients. Similar to working with medical interdisciplinary teams, when providing feedback at IEP meetings, it helps to keep information short and to the point.

o *I hit only the highlights, and I find it is helpful to tie findings back into the teacher's report. Bringing in a teacher's comments draws their attention to your findings and makes abstract cognitive concepts more relevant. "On the teacher form you wrote this ... you're probably seeing that because of these executive function issues I am talking about" (linking the test findings to the direct example in the teacher form).*

—Jennifer Janusz, Psy.D.

"Brain in a Bag" Technique for Communicating Findings to IEP Teams

IEP meetings can sometimes devolve into a dreaded war of standard scores ("Dr. Postal, you say here in your report Sally had a standard score of 85 on the processing speed task, but we have a standard score of 90....") A great technique to avoid this, and to bring the team conversation to a place where the child's brain function is connected to academic needs rather than a discussion of scores, is to bring a "brain in a bag." A classic, molded, 3D brain model fits nicely into a book bag, and can be pulled out as soon as one is invited to present one's findings.

o *"I always travel with my brain!" (Helps to start with some humor). "Actually, I brought this so we can talk about what's happening in Sally's brain." (Holds up model) "Here are the eyes, and this part of the brain is the frontal lobe. This part of the brain brings us all the functions we value in successful students. For example, the ability to drag attention from the most interesting thing in the room, towards their work. It also is involved in regulating mood and temper. What happened with the TBI a few months ago is that this part of the brain stopped working as well as it used to for Sally" (Or, "our testing showed Sally has ADHD, and this is the part of the brain most involved in this disorder"). "This is one reason that Sally is so distractible in math class. She can focus in art class really well because, to her, art is the most interesting thing in the room, but in math, which has always been the least interesting thing for her, that frontal system isn't working well enough to keep her focused. It also speaks to why her temper is blowing so often. Rather than 'talking her down,' like we would expect, her frontal system is letting those waves of emotion crest—and that's creating big disruptions. Let's talk about some strategies to help her frontal system do its job more efficiently."*

—Karen Postal, Ph.D.

COMMUNICATING WITH MILITARY COLLEAGUES

In a military setting, it is important to give feedback to patients' commanding officers. Typically, neuropsychologists will get permission from the patient, although the military rules regarding confidentiality are different from civilian rules. Special Forces commanders in particular, typically want to do whatever it takes to "preserve the asset." Concepts like "investment in soldier" are important priorities in the military, as is focusing on what will help the mission.

Feedback to commanders is usually in the form of a telephone conversation; this is often educational, where the effect of a TBI is discussed. Gender and civilian status play an important role in this conversation. With some Old Guard officers, females are given less respect. Of course, this can also be true for civilian personnel. Using military bearing during these conversations, including formal titles, is expected. Using specific military language like "asset" or using words like "stress" rather than "depression" or "anxiety" will increase the likelihood of one's message being heard.

> o *"Sir, Private Smith's neuropsychological assessment revealed.... Stress is a significant factor in prolonging his recovery. In order to protect this asset, we will need to...."*
>
> —*Laurie Ryan, Ph.D.*

The main point of military evaluations is to answer the question, "Can this patient continue to do his job?" The feedback to commanders is oriented to that question. For example, in a recent neuropsychological evaluation of an air traffic controller with dyslexia, the feedback session was about the need to retrain him for a different position.

Typically, feedback is given to the patient first and then given to the commanders and unit. However, if the patient seems like he might not handle the information well, then feedback might be communicated to the commander/unit first so they can be prepared to deal with him.

> o *"Sir, Sergeant Jones cannot continue to perform his job as an air traffic controller. He has dyslexia, and this interferes with his ability to rapidly process incoming data. He can retrain for another position. We have some data to share regarding his areas of strength...."*
>
> —*Laurie Ryan, Ph.D.*

Military settings consider personnel "assets," and part of the commander's job is to protect the assets to perform the mission. Invoking the concept of protecting assets can help non-medical officers understand the need to allow time off from training to recover even when the soldier looks physically fine.

> o *"Sir, this private has had a mild brain injury. The expected outcome is that he will recover fully, but he needs to rest over the next month. If he has time without" (list restrictions like no marching in 100 degree heat), "he should recover fully. If we don't give him time to recover, we might lose this asset."*
>
> —*Laurie Ryan, Ph.D.*

16 Report Writing and Written Communication

IN MOST CLINICAL practices, the written report is the primary means of communicating assessment results with other professionals. Given the complex nature of neuropsychological assessment findings, and the limited attention and memory capacity of many patients, effective written communication is also a means to enhance the feedback process. Just as the target audience of neuropsychological feedback has evolved to include patients rather than just our referring colleagues, the target audience of neuropsychological assessment reports has also evolved from writing exclusively to physicians, to now include patients, as well as a number of other professionals involved in the patient's life. Indeed, most clinicians told us that they either routinely send every patient a copy of their report, or they write the report assuming the patient will eventually read it.

A full discussion of neuropsychological report writing is beyond the scope of this book. However, as many of the clinicians we interviewed indicated that their written report was a natural extension of their feedback sessions, we conclude with some pearls regarding report writing.

TIMING OF REPORT DISTRIBUTION

The timing of reports is a matter of both philosophy and convenience. Clinicians generally describe utilizing one of five strategies: 1) send the report prior to the feedback session so patients and families can read it, offer corrections, and be prepared to ask questions; 2) simultaneously mail a rapid report to the patient and referring colleague to avoid any surprises should the patient meet with the referral source prior to the feedback session; 3) hand the report to the patient and/or family to follow during the feedback session; 4) give the report at the feedback session, but do not directly address the report during the appointment; or 5) integrate information from the feedback session into the final report and subsequently mail the completed version.

All of these approaches have their benefits and drawbacks. For example, sending the report after a feedback session, or even handing it to the family at the appointment, increases the likelihood that a clinician will have to deal with subsequent phone calls, clarifying questions, and requests for revisions. Similarly, mailing the report before a feedback session requires careful preparation of the patient and family as well as more foreshadowing of one's findings, especially if the differential diagnoses include topics such as mental retardation, dementia, or other conditions that carry significant emotional burdens. When families are not adequately prepared for the findings, it can lead to unnecessary, and even negative consequences. For example, one neuropsychologist told us, "I used to send the report to families ahead of time, but they very frequently did not understand it, and came to the feedback sessions angry."

On the other hand, under the right circumstances, and with the right families, receiving the report (or a draft of the report) ahead of time can lead to a much more collaborative feedback session.

> *I tell families during the diagnostic interview that they will receive the report before we meet. I invite them to read through the report and write all over it. I'll tell them, "be sure to mark any historical inaccuracies, and highlight any parts that you want to discuss or clarify. If the report includes information that seems incorrect or doesn't make sense, I will count on you to tell me that when we meet. That*

way you will be able to walk away with all of your questions answered, and with a corrected/updated report." I also warn parents, "If I'm concerned that your child is not getting enough services at school, I'll spend a great deal of time emphasizing your child's weaknesses. I'll talk about the strengths, but it's usually in a single, relatively small, paragraph. So, if the report seems overwhelming, put it away. I promise that when you leave the feedback session, you'll be saying to yourself, 'Oh I knew all that,' because you already know your child better than anyone else."

I also typically share with parents my initial impressions at the end of the testing session(s). Consequently, they are never provided with a diagnostic conclusion in writing that they have not already heard in person, even though they get the report before our feedback session.

—*Kira Armstrong, Ph.D.*

Amongst those who have a copy of the report ready at the feedback session, some give it to families immediately and read through the report together.

When patients return for feedback, I begin the session by giving them a copy of the evaluation report. I bring their attention to the Summary and Recommendations section and read this section aloud. I invite them to read along with each paragraph. I pause and try to clarify any questions they may have or issues they may not understand. I tell them, "There's a lot of words in this report that may be difficult to understand, such as specific test findings. The most important point is that when you leave this office, you understand the summary and recommendations."

—*Julie Bobholz, Ph.D.*

Cheryl Weinstein gives families a copy of the report that she describes as "a draft."

o *I don't want them looking at the rest of the report and saying, "she made those errors in history—I don't trust the rest of the report." So, I hand the draft report to the families and say, "Look at the history, tell me what's incorrect? Take a red pen, anywhere in the report, things that you don't agree with. Come back in a month, and we will sit down again and discuss the report and recommendations."*

Others hand the report to families at the feedback session for future reference. For example, Michael Westerveld tells parents:

o *"The testing doesn't do you any good unless you can use it and understand it. The report is something that you can refer back to later so it can remind you about what we talked about during the feedback. But that's not what we are going to focus on today. Today's feedback is to answer your questions and understand what is in the report when you refer to it later."*

Christopher Nicholls also hands the report to families at the end of the feedback session, noting:

o *"Look, we've talked about a lot of information. Take this home, read it, and if you have questions, come back and we can talk again."*

Finally, many clinicians incorporate data gathered from the feedback session into their report, and then send out a copy a week or so later. Misunderstandings regarding symptom course, aspects of the history, or feasibility of recommendations might surface at feedback, and these can be corrected prior to becoming part of the medical record. Often, patients and families will resonate with specific findings and bring up additional clinical data that create a richer final report.

PROVIDING HANDOUTS AND WRITTEN SUMMARIES AT THE FEEDBACK SESSION

If a report is not available at the feedback session, many neuropsychologists will prepare a written handout for patients. This typically includes a very brief summary of test findings, bullet-point diagnoses, and recommendations. This practice not only serves as a useful reference point for the patient and family, it is also an excellent way for students or early-career neuropsychologists to clarify and organize their thinking prior to sitting down with families.

Karen Wills hands families and patients a one-page bullet-point summary. She tries to distill the information into three main issues, couched in positive terms (e.g., Normal IQ and academic achievement on untimed tests … lower scores on timed tests … he did great on visual abstract reasoning). She then prioritizes the recommendations and breaks them down into discrete domains: medical, education, and psychosocial. Likewise, Gerry Taylor writes out recommendations prior to feedback sessions and hands them to parents to take with them. These recommendations can also be given to the school. Finally, Bernice Marcopulos and her peers hand psychiatric inpatients a brochure that describes the testing they participated in, and has a fill-in-the-blank section, where clinicians briefly describe the findings and treatment recommendations in simple, clear language. When we think of our patients as our customers, this practice is literally allowing them to leave our offices with what they came for.

Robin Hanks points out that, even if you don't have a cognitive impairment, remembering all of the information given to you after a doctor's appointment can be challenging. It helps patients to have something concrete to take with them, like a written summary of findings from the neuropsychological report written in lay terms.

> *They are then less likely to ask for a copy of their report. They want to know the results and recommendations—they don't care what the individual scores were, or tests given. They want the outcome.*

LENGTH OF REPORTS

As a teaching tool for nascent neuropsychologists, lengthy reports allow supervisors to clearly observe and critique students' reasoning and knowledge. As a tool of medical communication, particularly in the context of neurology referrals or interdisciplinary teams, lengthy reports can be a liability. Aaron Nelson points out that when he reads reports by people in our guild that are 20 to 30 pages long, with each test completely factor-analyzed, it often appears as though the clinician does not know what they are doing. Likewise, Erin

Bigler declares that lengthy reports with pages of conclusions "are absolutely worthless." He requires his students to write short reports of no more than two to five pages. He also emphasizes that:

> My goal is to keep the neuropsychology service focused on neurological problems. The neurologist wants a brief statement. Is this person demented? Can they go home and deal with ADLs? I'll ask my students, "Can you say this in three sentences or less? If not, go back and rethink."

Robert Heilbronner also writes a short report with an annotated history when his patents are referred from an adult neurology practice.

> I typically don't repeat everything that's already been done. In some regard the neuropsychological report is the opportunity to integrate everything. But my clinical reports simply state, "You are familiar with Mr. Smith's history. The following is important to note as it relates to his neurocognitive status.... " Then I include the tests administered, cognitive and emotional functions sections, summary, and recommendations.

Some clinicians offer even shorter reports, especially when they are working on a multidisciplinary team.

> My reports are very short, about 1½ pages. I don't communicate any scores. I provide a brief referral reason, background, behavioral observations, findings (without scores), and a paragraph on concerns and goals.
>
> —Cynthia Kubu, Ph.D.

Of course, some neuropsychologists write longer reports, and this choice is often dictated, at least in part, by the kind of clinical practice and referral sources with which one works. For example, forensic settings typically demand a longer, more inclusive report writing strategy, and are beyond the scope of this book. Pediatric neuropsychologists also tend to write longer reports, particularly when communicating with parents and IEP teams. Longer reports typically include an integration of relevant history and previous assessments (which in pediatric cases might rival the paperwork of a civil legal case). Many clinicians who write longer reports also make an effort to include consumer-friendly language to help translate some of the many "jargon" terms used by our profession.

> I use a lot of lay language in my reports. For example, I will describe Logical Memory I and II from the Wechsler Memory Scale-IV, as a memory test that is similar to hearing and retaining information from a conversation.
>
> —Susan McPherson, Ph.D.

Consumer-oriented reports are not necessarily helpful in all settings or for all clinicians. Aaron Nelson comments,

> Patients are entitled to a copy of the report. What they are not entitled to is neuropsychology lessons. Having a chest X-ray does not buy you an explanation of the physics of photons from the radiologist who read the film. The neuropsychological

evaluation report is an archival record intended for medical use. I want patients to come away from the encounter with a full understanding of what my thoughts are and the opportunity to have their questions answered as satisfactorily as possible. But for example, if someone were to ask me, "What does this code type mean on this test, MMPI? What is a code type?" I don't feel the compulsion to give them a course on psychometric theory. So I'll tell them, "Those are technical issues—what's important is my impression...."

KNOWING YOUR AUDIENCE

The decision to write longer or shorter reports, to include jargon or more user-friendly language, or to simply provide brief summaries of the findings is often dictated by an awareness of who will be receiving the information. Longer reports with more explanations may indeed be better received by patients and their families, but medical professionals (i.e., referral sources) are often interested in a much quicker summary of the findings.

A number of years ago a neurologist referred a large number of patients to me. When we met for the first time he said, "Ted, I love your reports, but unless you make a change, I will stop referring to you. I archive all old records on microfiche. It costs me a certain amount of money per page. Unless you cut it down, I will refer to someone else. I don't care if you write a long report—keep it in your own chart. All I want is a one- to two- page executive summary. I don't even look at all that other stuff."

—Edward Ted Peck, Ph.D.

Based on this feedback, Ted Peck and his colleagues revised their approach to reports, and now rely on a more streamlined model:

Our practice prides itself on our prompt reports—within a week of seeing the patient. If you are going to follow a medical model of service, you need to get results promptly back to physicians. You do not have the luxury of taking a month or two months to write a report, or the luxury of writing 10-page reports. Our reports are two to three and a half pages, although some pediatric reports contain an extra page. These include a brief history, report data, interpretation, and diagnosis.

With the history section, I dictate only two to three sentences, such as, "Eight-year history of MS, relapsing remitting. The past medical history is noted elsewhere in the chart." I do not dictate a multi-page history. I'll include a statement of "History is positive for:" and include only what is relevant to the referral source. For example, if the referral is about memory, there is no need to include a left femur fracture 25 years ago. Multiple concussions would be relevant, though.

Others take steps to meet the needs of both the medical professionals and patients. For example, some clinicians will write relatively lengthy reports, and attach a one- to two-page cover letter summarizing the primary findings. This gives readers the "best of both worlds:" the opportunity to cut to the chase, and to develop a more comprehensive understanding of the neuropsychological findings, conclusions, and recommendations.

REMEMBERING THE POWER OF THE WRITTEN WORD

Marla Shapiro tries never to forget, as she goes about the routine business of writing reports, that these reports are anything but routine for our clients. She emphasizes that we need to always remember just how potent and emotionally charged our words can be. She tells this story to trainees and students when they talk about report writing.

> When I was starting my pre-doctoral internship, I co-led a group for parents of children with TBI, to help them use our neuropsych evaluation results to better understand their kids' day-to-day behaviors. The first task of the group was to actually find, and bring in their most recent evaluation report. One mom just kept forgetting. We even gave her a new copy of the report, and she still forgot it. So, one week, we asked her why. She told us that she brought it home, put it on the kitchen counter where she walked past it every day, and it just sat there like a snake waiting to bite her. She knew what it said and had few illusions left about her child, but seeing it there in black and white, staring at her from the page … well, it was like a snake just sitting there and waiting to bite her.

This is an excellent reminder of the fact that even when a patient or family member fully understands their cognitive strengths and weaknesses, sometimes seeing this information laid out in writing makes everything so much more "real," and at times that much more painful. Providing this information in the context of an empathetic, supportive feedback session, however, can be the first step in helping the patient and family accept the findings and move forward.

Similarly, Margaret O'Connor frequently reminds her students to be careful about how they describe patients:

> Students have often been taught to comment on individuals' physical features, and they may describe people as having "funny faces," as "obese," or "looking older than their years." There are times when these comments are clinically relevant, but there are times when they are not needed, and they can be quite offensive. I don't think that students understand how invasive our evaluations are. Even more experienced clinicians can become desensitized to this (so a reminder now and then can be important for them, too).
>
> —Margaret O'Connor, Ph.D.

Explaining this concept to her students is not quite enough. Dr. O'Connor also takes the time to ensure that her patients are able to recognize the difference between describing their condition and describing them as a person:

> o During the feedback session I read the reports aloud to the patient. Before doing so I often say, "This may be the first time in your adult life that you've heard yourself described on paper. I want you to know this is not what I think of you as a person. This is a problem-oriented evaluation, so we're going to talk about some of the issues that you brought to the table that are difficult for you."
>
> —Margaret O'Connor, Ph.D.

Epilogue

KAREN WILLS RECALLS BYRON Rourke summing up the complex nature of our field beautifully: "Neuropsychology is total psychology. Everything you have ever learned about child development, family therapy, psychopathology, testing, evaluation, communication skills, and life in general. There is nothing you have learned in your entire life that won't be important, and you will use it all at once. This is the coolest and most complicated thing you will ever do."

We hope that this book provides one more resource for clinicians to communicate all of their nuanced findings with patients, families, and other professionals. We also hope that this book stimulates ideas, discussion, and further research about how to effectively provide feedback in the context of neuropsychological assessment.

Printed in the USA/Agawam, MA
September 21, 2018

683633.002